THE ULTIMATE INSTANT POT COOKBOOK

by

Joe Boardman

Published by

Starzend Publishing

Des Moines, IA

The Ultimate Instant Pot Cookbook

by Joe Boardman

Published by Starzend Publishing

Des Moines, IA

First Printing: November 9, 2018

Print:

ISBN-13/EAN-13: 978-1793-12-9

Printed in the United States of America

THE ULTIMATE INSTANT POT COOKBOOK

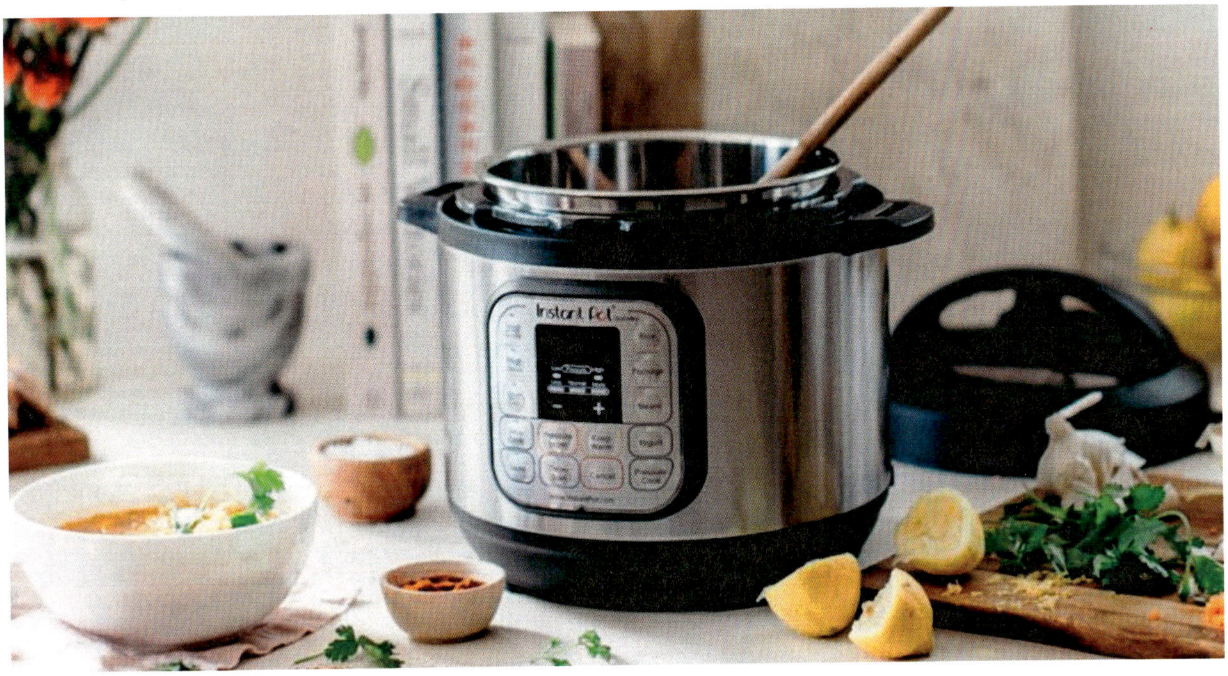

INTRODUCTION

Cooking just got a whole lot smarter with Instant Pots. This multi-tasking device is designed to make cooking easier and more convenient. Instant Pots features a variety of different functions such as steaming, stewing, roasting and baking. In addition, you can sauté/sear, cook rice, warm and slow cook in your Instant Pot. Instant Pot has built-in smart programs; with a simple push of a button all your favorite dishes are cooked to perfection. The best part about using Instant Pot is that the inner pot is dishwasher safe. Cleaning up is just as easy and quick as your meal prep.

Not sure where to start?

- Pressure cooking is the primary function of instant pot; it’s also the reason why the Instant Pot is a versatile cooking appliance. Using both pressure and heat, Instant pot can prepare food quickly and evenly. Pressure cooking retains your food's nutrients and flavors while creating delicious results. The cooking process usually takes half the time on an Instant Pot saving energy in the process.
- Slow cooking. The Instant Pot has a slow cook function for long and gentle cooking. It's more convenient to cook food slowly sometimes.

- Steams and sauté. The Instant Pot has a built-in heat source at the base; this means you can use the pot to simmer liquids for steaming, sauté vegetables and sear meats.
- Rice cooker. With the Instant Pot, you can make rice easily with just a touch of a button. You can also use your Instant Pot to make Yogurt.

SETTING UP YOUR INSTANT POT

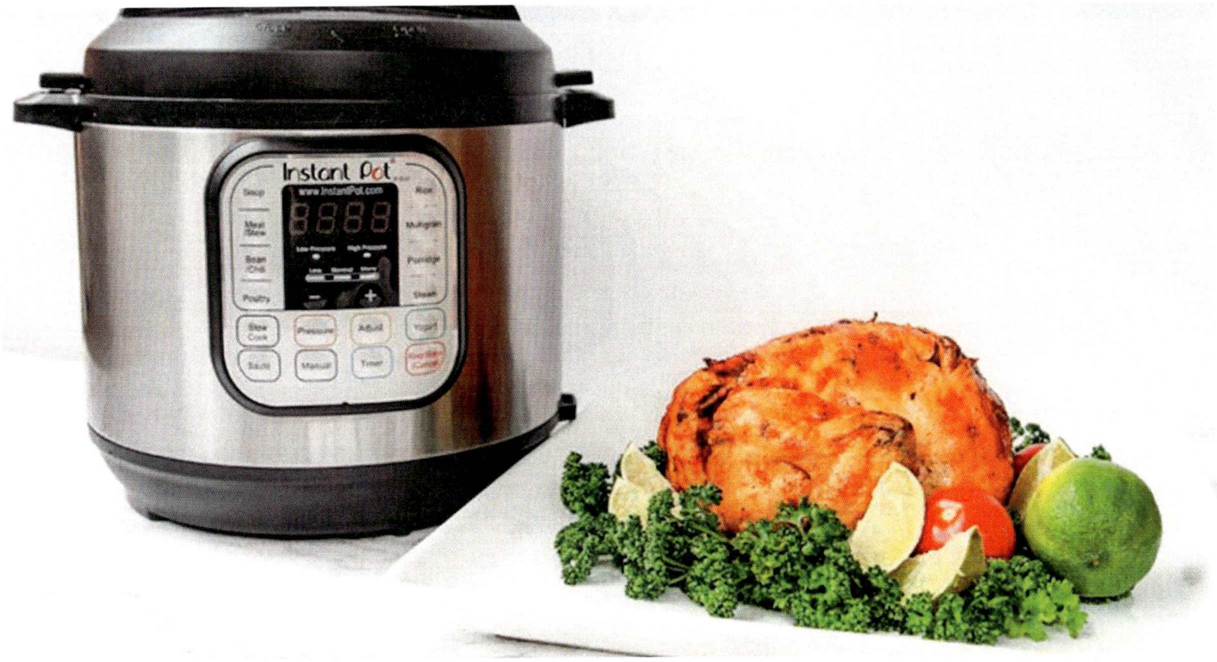

Now that you have an idea of what your multi-cooker can do, it's time to set it up and find out what parts it comes with and any additional accessories you might need. The most important part of the Instant Pot is the electrical cord, plug the cord into the pot. Other accessories include:

Inner pot

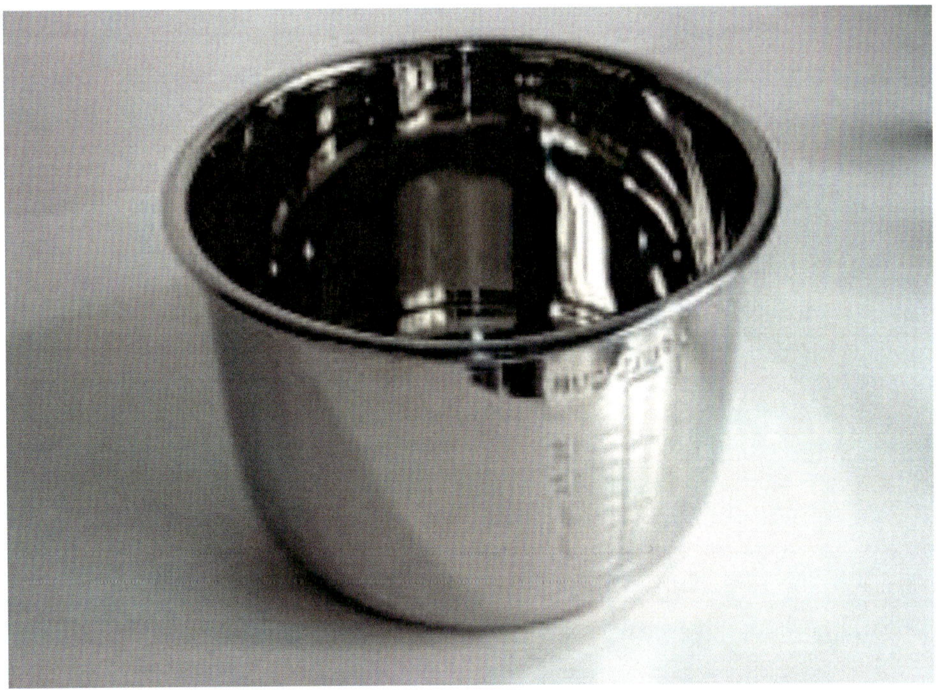

Inner pot – food cooks in the inner pot which is usually nonstick or stainless steel. You should remove the inner pot regularly for cleaning. Other than the Inner Pot you can use other oven-safe utensils to cook. Use a springform pan to bake, the little 6" or 7" perfectly fits in the Instant Pot. Silicon cupcake liners also come in handy when making mini cakes, eggs and more.

Get Instant Pot mini mitts; you don't want to get burned every time you deal with these hot attachments.

Steam rack trivet/steam basket

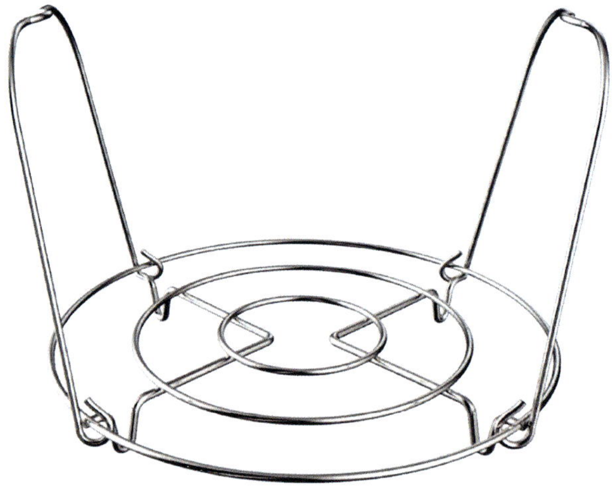

Steam rack trivet/steam basket– the steaming rack or basket sits in the inner pot, and it comes in handy for when you don't want your food submerged. It keeps your food raised above the liquid. Some foods and small vegetables usually fall through the steam rack to avoid this problem place the steam basket on top of the steam rack.

Condensation collector

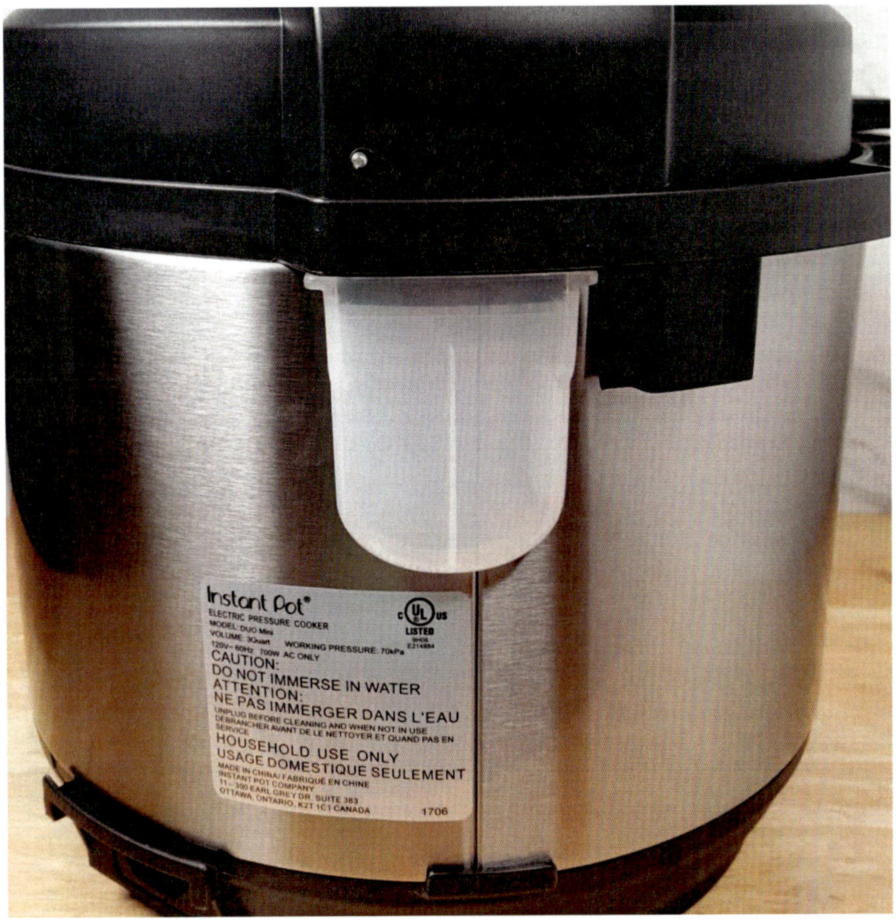

Condensation Collector – it's a small plastic cup that hooks onto the outer body of the Instant Pot and keeps the condensation from hitting the counter during slow cooking and cooling. Slide the condensation collector onto the pot's side, and it should click into place.

Pot lid

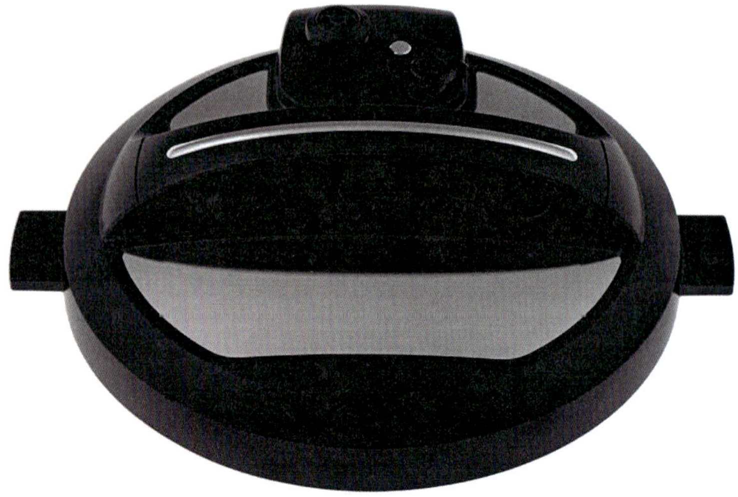

Pot lid – the lid of the Instant Pot is an integral part of the multi-cooker. You can't cook foods under pressure without the lid. The lid keeps the steam in the pot, and it needs to be locked in place before turning on the pressure-cooking function. Some Instant Pots have detachable lids while others the lid is secured to the outer body.

Steam Release Valve

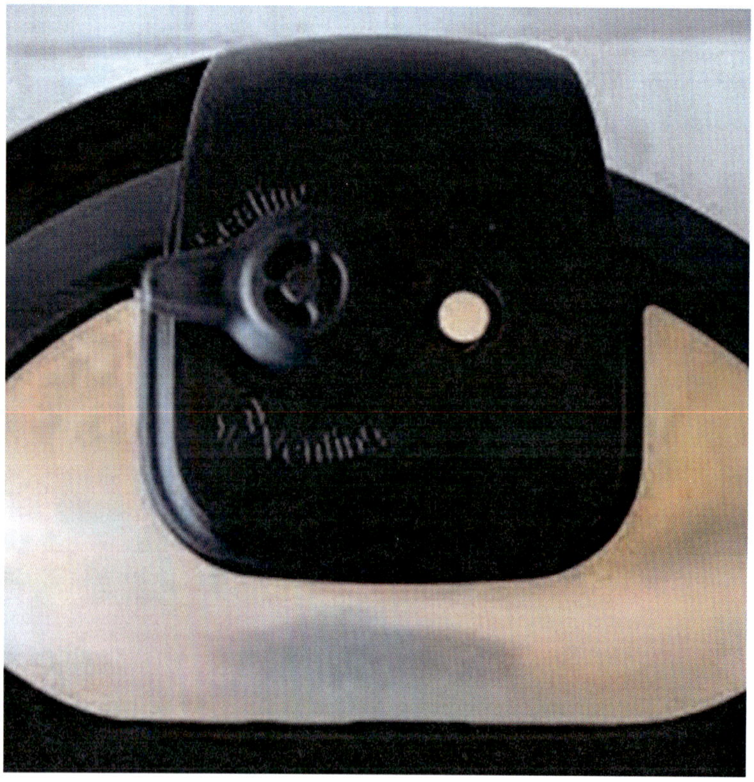

Steam release valve – the steam valve is found on the pot's lid; the valve allows pressure to build in the pot or release it. Basically, the valve has to setting, sealing and venting. The valve should be in sealing (locked) position when using the pressure-cooking function. The valve should be in Venting (open) position when using the slow cooking function.

How to release pressure

There are two ways to release the built-up pressure once the Instant Pot cooker completes its cooking cycle.

- Quick Release – you will want to immediately stop cooking foods that have a quick cook time. Do a quick release by pushing the valve on the pot lid from sealing setting to venting setting. After the steam release from the pot and the pressure valve has dropped to the lowest position and venting has stopped you can safely open the pot.
- Natural Release – the pot naturally begins to release steam after the programmed time is over if you don't do a Quick Release. Pressure naturally dissipates on its own, and it usually takes between 10-20 minutes depending on how long your food has been cooking.

Sealing ring and Anti-block shield

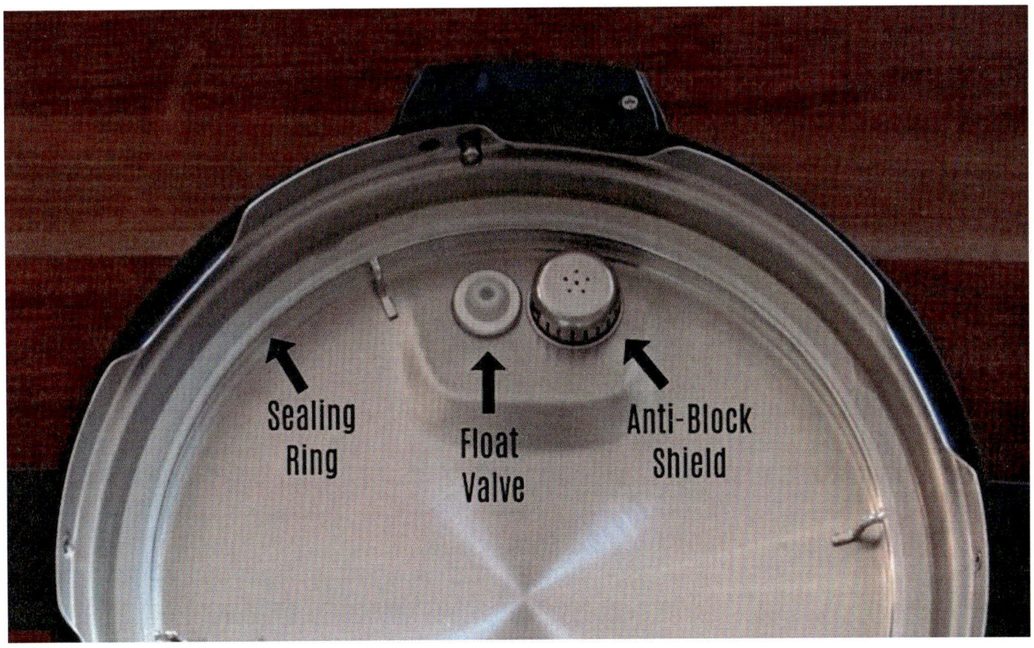

Sealing ring – this white silicone ring surrounds the lid. It seals steam into the pot allowing pressure to safely build in the pot. Sealing rings may retain odor from strongly scented foods like onions, garlic and ginger during the cooking process. Keep an extra sealing in hand for delicate dishes like custards, yogurt, mildly flavored desserts or plain rice. Always clean the sealing ring after use.

Anti-block shield – it prevents the foam generated during the cooking process and small foods from clogging the pressure release valve resulting in an unsafe amount of pressure to build-up. Always use the anti-block shield.

USING THE INSTANT POT

Never fill more than half of the pot when pressure cooking with the Instant Pot. Hot liquid might spray out of the pressure release valve if the pot contains too much liquid. Never fill the pot to the maximum level when pressure cooking as food usually expand under intense heat/pressure it might result in a safety problem. Only fill the pot to the maximum level when using slow cooker, rice cooker functions etc.

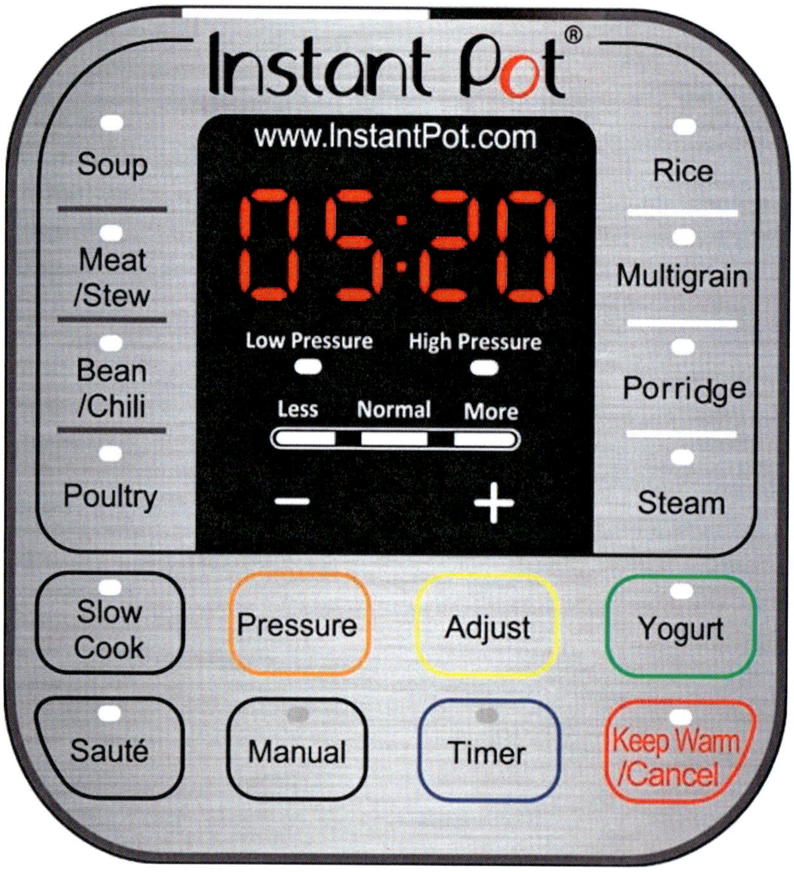

Usually, the Instant Pot has 16 settings. Each button on the control panel is designated to a specific type of cooking. These buttons have preset cook times to make the cooking process on the Instant Pot, easier, convenient as well as eliminate guesswork. The settings on the button also help you to know whether the pot will be in a pressure-cooking setting or slow cooker setting which cooks without pressure.

Instant Pot Cooking Guide

COOKING GUIDE

Cooking Function	Default Setting	Pressure Adjustments	Temperature Adjustments	Cook Time Range
SLOW COOK	High temp / 4 hours	N/A	Low-High	30 minutes – 20 hours
STEAM	High pressure / 10 minutes	Low-High	N/A	3 minutes – 1 hour
BROWN/ SAUTÉ	High temp / 30 minutes	N/A	Low-High	5 minutes – 30 minutes
KEEP WARM	Warm temp / 4 hours	N/A	Warm	30 minutes – 4 hours
MEAT/STEW	High pressure / 35 minutes	Low-High	N/A	15 minutes – 2 hours
BEANS/CHILI	High pressure / 20 minutes	Low-High	N/A	5 minutes – 2 hours
RICE/ RISOTTO	Low pressure / 12 minutes	Low-High	N/A	6 minutes – 30 minutes
YOGURT	Low temp / 8 hours	N/A	Low-High	Low: 6 hours - 12 hours High: N/A
POULTRY	High pressure / 15 minutes	Low-High	N/A	15 minutes – 2 hours
DESSERT	Low pressure / 10 minutes	Low-High	N/A	5 minutes – 2 hours
SOUP	High pressure / 30 minutes	Low-High	N/A	5 minutes – 2 hours
MULTIGRAIN	High pressure / 40 minutes	Low-High	N/A	10 minutes – 2 hours

"High Pressure" setting indicates that the Instant Pot is cooking at high pressure and the lid is sealed while the "Low Pressure" setting indicates the Instant Pot low pressure cooking and the "Normal" setting shows the Instant Pot is working as a slow cooker and it's not using pressure or sealed.

Instant Pot Cooking Cheat Sheet

Cooking Charts

	Cooking Time HIGH pressure (minutes)	Liquid Needed	Release Method		Cooking Time HIGH pressure (minutes)	Liquid Needed	Release Method
Poultry							
Chicken Bones for stock	40	6 cups	NATURAL	Chicken Thigh (boneless)	4	1 cup	QUICK
Chicken Breast (bone in)	6	1 cup	QUICK	Chicken, Whole	20	1½ cups	NATURAL
Chicken Breast (boneless)	4	1 cup	QUICK	Cornish Game Hen (1 to 1½ pounds)	8	1 cup	NATURAL
Chicken Thigh (bone in)	7	1 cup	QUICK	Turkey Breast (boneless, 2 to 3 pounds)	20 to 25	1½ cups	NATURAL
Beef							
Beef Bones for stock	40	6 cups	NATURAL	Meatloaf	35	1½ cups	NATURAL
Brisket (3½ to 4 pounds)	55 to 65	1½ cups	NATURAL	Pot Roast (3½ to 4 pounds)	55 to 65	2 cups	NATURAL
Corned Beef Brisket	55	covered	NATURAL	Short Ribs	55	1½ cups	NATURAL
Flank Steak (1 pound)	25	1 cup	NATURAL	Stew Meat (1-inch cubes)	15 to 20	1 cup	NATURAL
Ground Beef	5	1 cup	QUICK	Veal Shanks	20 to 25	1½ cups	NATURAL
Meatballs	5	1 cup	NATURAL	Veal Stew Meat (1-inch cubes)	10	1 cup	NATURAL
Pork							
Baby Back Ribs	30	1 cup	NATURAL	Pork Chops (boneless, 1-inch)	4 to 5	1½ cups	NATURAL
Country Style Ribs	20 to 25	1½ cups	NATURAL	Pork Loin (2 to 2½ pounds)	25	1½ cups	NATURAL
Ground Pork	5	1 cup	QUICK	Pork Shoulder (3 pounds)	55	1½ cups	NATURAL
Ham (bone in, 5 pounds, pre-cooked)	25 to 30	1½ cups	NATURAL	Sausages	10 to 15	1½ cups	QUICK
				Spare Ribs	45	1 cup	NATURAL
Meatballs	5	1 cup	NATURAL	Stew Meat (1-inch cubes)	15 to 20	1 cup	NATURAL
Pork Chops (bone in, 1-inch)	6	1½ cups	NATURAL				
Lamb							
Ground Lamb	5	1 cup	QUICK	Leg of Lamb (boneless, 3½ to 4 pounds)	35 to 45	1½ cups	NATURAL
Lamb Shanks	30	1½ cups	NATURAL	Stew Meat (1-inch cubes)	15 to 20	1 cup	NATURAL
Meatballs	5	1 cup	NATURAL				
Fish and Seafood							
Calamari	20	5 cup	QUICK	Mussels	4	2 cup	QUICK
Clams	4	1 cup	QUICK	Salmon	5	4 cup	QUICK
Crab Legs	4	1 cup	QUICK	Shrimp	2	3 cup	QUICK
Fish Fillet (1-inch thick)	5	6 cup	QUICK				

Cooking Charts

	Cooking Time HIGH pressure (minutes)	Liquid Needed	Release Method		Cooking Time HIGH pressure (minutes)	Liquid Needed	Release Method
Grains (1 cup)							
Barley (pearled)	20 to 25	3 cups	QUICK	Poletna (fine, not instant)	5	4 cups	QUICK
Brown Rice	20	2 cups	NATURAL	Quinoa	5	1½ cups	QUICK
Bulgur	6	2 cups	QUICK	Steel Cut Oats	5	3 cups	NATURAL
Farro (pearled)	8	2 cups	QUICK	White Rice, long-grain	4 to 6	1½ cups	QUICK
Farro (whole grain)	18	3 cups	QUICK	White Rice, short-grain	7	2⅔ cups	QUICK
Polenta (coarse, not instant)	8 to 10	4 cups	QUICK	Wild Rice	22	3 to 4 cups	QUICK
Beans and Legumes							
	Un-Soaked	Soaked or Quick-Soaked			Un-Soaked	Soaked or Quick-Soaked	
Black Beans	25	7	NATURAL	Kidney Beans	25	8 to 10	NATURAL
Black-Eyed Peas	8	6	NATURAL	Lentils	7 to 8	unnecessary	QUICK
Cannellini Beans	25	7	NATURAL	Navy Beans	20	8 to 10	NATURAL
Chickpeas	35 to 40	15	NATURAL	Pinto Beans	25	8 to 10	NATURAL
Great Northern Beans	25	8 to 10	NATURAL	Split Peas	8 to 10	unnecessary	NATURAL
				White Beans	20	8 to 10	NATURAL
Vegetables							
Acorn Squash (halved)	8	1 cup	QUICK	Eggplant	3 to 4	1 cup	QUICK
Artichokes (medium, whole)	12	1 cup	QUICK	Fennel (wedges)	4	1 cup	QUICK
Asparagus	2	1 cup	QUICK	Green Beans	3 to 4	1 cup	QUICK
Beets (medium, whole)	15	1 cup	QUICK	Kale	4	1 cup	QUICK
Broccoli	3	1 cup	QUICK	Leeks (1-inch pieces)	4	1 cup	QUICK
Broccoli Rabe	3	1 cup	QUICK	Parsnips (1-inch chunks)	4 to 5	1 cup	QUICK
Brussels Sprouts	4 to 6	1 cup	QUICK	Potatoes (1-inch chunks or small whole)	6 to 8	1 cup	QUICK
Butternut Squash (1-inch cubes)	5	1 cup	QUICK	Rutabaga (1-inch chunks)	4	1 cup	QUICK
Cabbage (quartered)	4 to 6	1 cup	QUICK	Spaghetti Squash (halved)	12 to 15	1 cup	QUICK
Beets (medium, whole)	15	1 cup	QUICK	Sweet Potatoes (1-inch chunks)	4 to 5	1 cup	QUICK
Cauliflower (whole)	12 to 15	1 cup	QUICK	Swiss Chard	2	1 cup	QUICK
Collard Greens	5 to 10	1 cup	QUICK	Turnips (1-inch chunks)	3 to 4	1 cup	QUICK
Corn on the Cob	2 to 3	1 cup	QUICK				

KEEP WARM FUNCTION

The "Keep Warm" function will automatically turn on when the timer goes off indicating that cooking is done.

INITIAL TEST RUN

You are now ready for an initial test run of your Instant Pot. An initial test run is the best way to test the Instant Pot and give you the confidence to get started in the wonderful world of Instant Pots.

- Ensure that the sealing ring is properly aligned with the lid, the float valve and the steam release handle are unobstructed.
- Also, ensure that the steam release handle and float valve are unobstructed. The sealing ring should always be properly aligned with the lid.
- Add water up to the "3" mark in the inner pot.
- Press the pre-set steam button.
- Press the minus (-) sign to change the time to 2 minutes
- The Instant Pot will be in pre-heating cycle after 10 seconds. Steam will release out of the valve within minutes. After a while, the float valve will pop up and seal the cooker.
- A beep will go off signaling the timer has finished the countdown. The Instant Pot goes automatically into "Keep Warm" mode after the timer goes off.
- You can choose to either do a Quick Release (as explained above) or wait for the Instant Pot to complete a Natural Release. Wait for about 10 minutes before pushing the vent valve and opening the lid.

QUICK TIPS

- As with any appliance ensure that you carefully read through the user manual before you begin using you Instant Pot.
- You don't have to defrost your frozen foods before cooking them in the Instant Pot.
- Always set the venting knob before pressing on a cooking function.
- Use aluminum foil to clean leftover residue.

Table of Contents

BREAKFAST

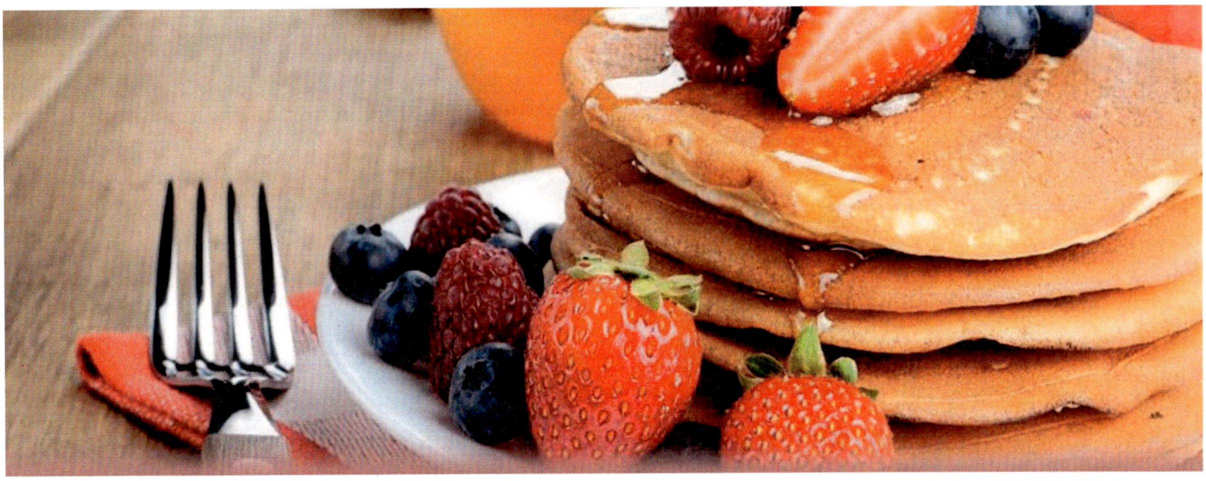

Breakfast is the first meal taken after a long night's sleep and often referred as the day's most important meal. However, some morning all we can do is grab a crappy granola bar or a fistful of cereal on our way out. A healthy balanced breakfast provides your brain and body with energy after the overnight fast. A healthy breakfast is a source of essential nutrients such as protein, vitamin B, calcium, iron, fiber for the body's needs. With all that preparing a daily gourmet breakfast is just an unrealistic goal. Instant Pot provides a perfect solution. It's amazing the number of healthy breakfast ideas you can make with little effort on your Instant Pot. From easy recipes that you can whip up within minutes to healthy recipes that you can make ahead of time here are healthy Instant Pot Breakfast recipes.

Lemon Blueberry Breakfast Cake

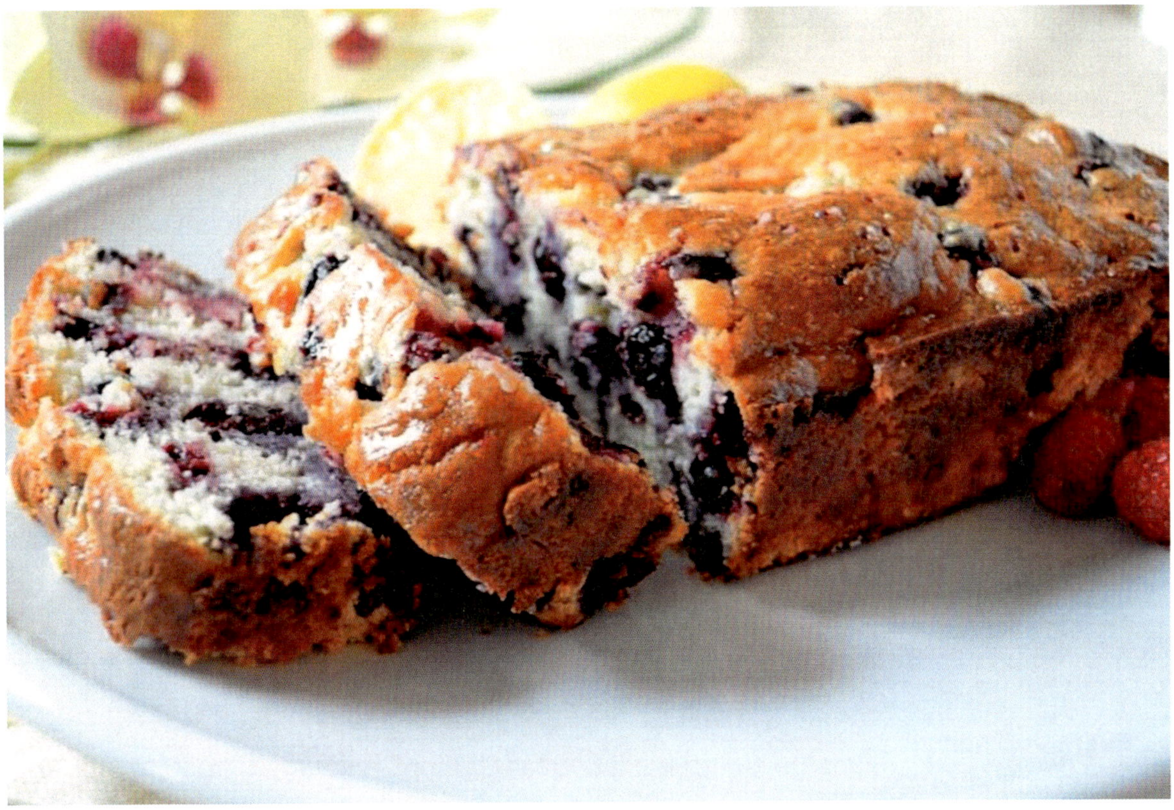

Prep Time: 20 minutes. Cook Time: 30 minutes. Total Time: 50 minutes.

Lemon Blueberry Breakfast Cake is an easy and quick breakfast meal. Just set it in your Instant Pot and carry on with your morning routine. Lemon Blueberry Breakfast Cake is also perfect for brunches.

Servings: 2

Ingredient

2 cups of all-purpose flour
2 teaspoons of baking powder
¾ cup of sugar
1 lemon zest
1 teaspoon vanilla extract
½ teaspoon of salt
½ cup of unsalted butter (room temperature)
½ cup buttermilk (or add a tablespoon of lemon juice in any milk)
1 egg
2 cups frozen or fresh blueberries

Optional

½ cup of powdered sugar
½ lemon juice

Instructions

1. Choose an appropriately sized dish for the Instant Pot.
2. Grease and flour the dish.
3. Mix the salt, baking powder and flour in a small bowl.
4. Add butter, zest and sugar into the mixer. Mix until the mixture is roughly combined. Finally add the egg and vanilla to the mixture.
5. Adding a cup at a time, pour your flour mixture and buttermilk into the mixture in the stand mixer.
6. Toss the blueberries lightly and gently fold into the batter.
7. Place the steam rack in the Instant Pot and add 2/3 cup of water. Place the batter into the floured and greased dish and place the dish in the Instant Pot.
8. Set the Instant Pot to "Manual" function and set the timer for 30 minutes.
9. Quick Release pressure when the timer goes off and remove the cake immediately. Transfer the cake to a serving dish after the condensation dissipates.
10. Mix ½ cup of powdered sugar and the juice from the ½ lemon for the cake glaze.
11. Serve and enjoy!

Quinoa Breakfast Bowl

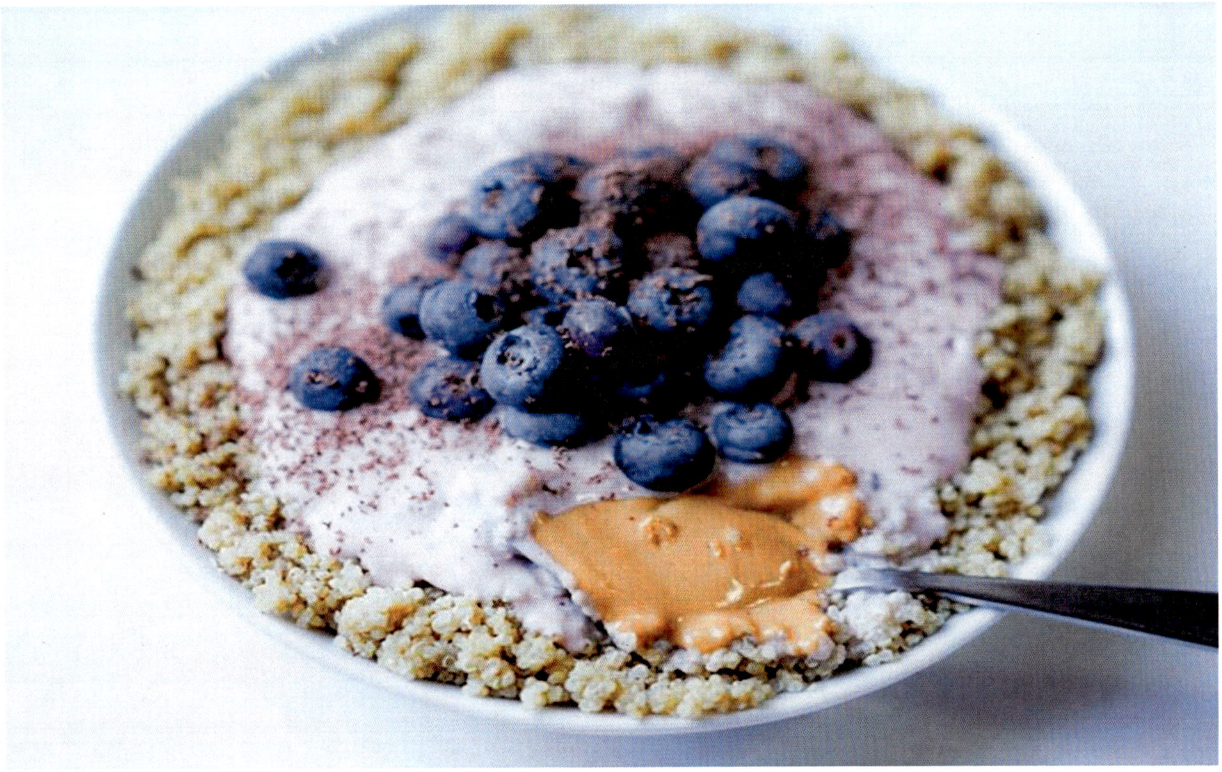

Prep Time: 25 minutes. Cook Time: 1 minute. Total Time: 26 minutes.

Quinoa breakfast bowl is an easy and healthy make-ahead breakfast recipe. It's a nutritious alternative to store-bought cereal. Quinoa only cooks for a minute in the Instant Pot.

Servings: 4

Ingredients

1½ cups quinoa soaked for at least an hour in water
1½ cups of water
1 can of coconut milk (or your milk of choice)
¼ cup maple syrup
2 teaspoons vanilla extract
1 teaspoon ground cinnamon
¼ teaspoon salt

Toppings (optional)

Non-dairy milk
Fresh fruit
Hemp hearts

Instructions

1. Rinse and drain the soaked quinoa and place it in a bowl. Add water, coconut milk, maple syrup, vanilla, cinnamon and salt into the bowl before transferring it into the Instant Pot. Seal the pot's lid, shut the vent and press the "Rice" setting. Once the timer goes off, allow Natural Pressure Release for around 10 minutes before opening the vent and removing the Instant Pot lid.
2. Divided the cooked quinoa into 6 individual containers containing about a cup of quinoa. Store the containers in the fridge. Quinoa can be preserved for a week in the fridge.
3. Add different toppings for each quinoa breakfast bowl.
4. Enjoy!

Mini-Frittata

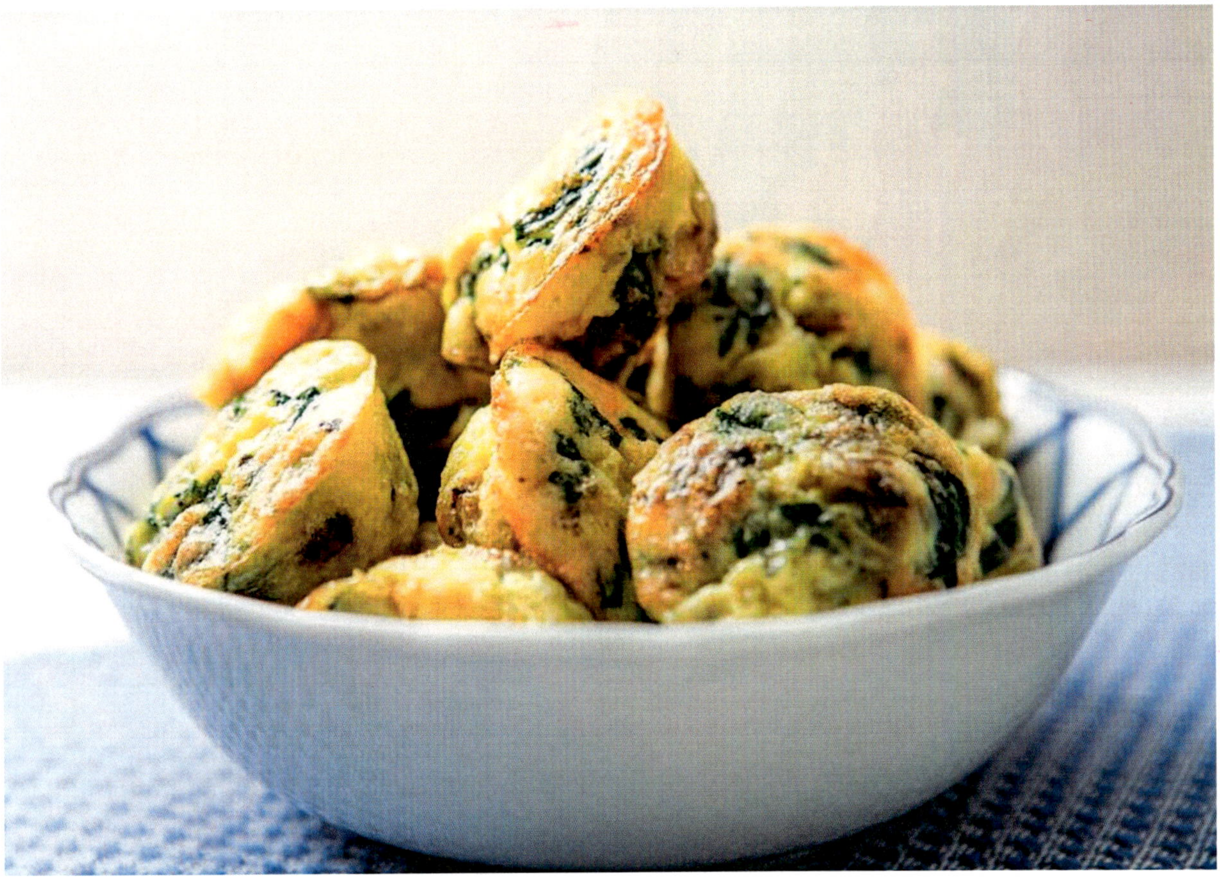

Prep time: 5 minutes. Cook time: 5 minutes. Total time: 10 minutes.

Mini-frittatas are easy and delicious to make in an Instant Pot. You can easily customize this recipe by elevating it or make it more kid-friendly.

Servings: 6

Ingredients

A splash of milk.
5 eggs
Salt and pepper

Mix in (Optional)

Meats
Veggies
Cheese

Instructions

1. Add milk, eggs and your choice of mix-ins in a mixing bowl. Stir the ingredients into a mixture.
2. Pour this mixture into individual baking molds.
3. Add a cup of water into the Instant Pot and place your molds on the steam rack.

4. Set the Instant Pot to "Manual" function and cook at "High Pressure" for about 5 minutes.
5. Do a Quick Release after the Instant Pot timer goes off. Carefully open the lid and remove the baking molds.
6. Serve and enjoy!

Bacon and Egg Risotto

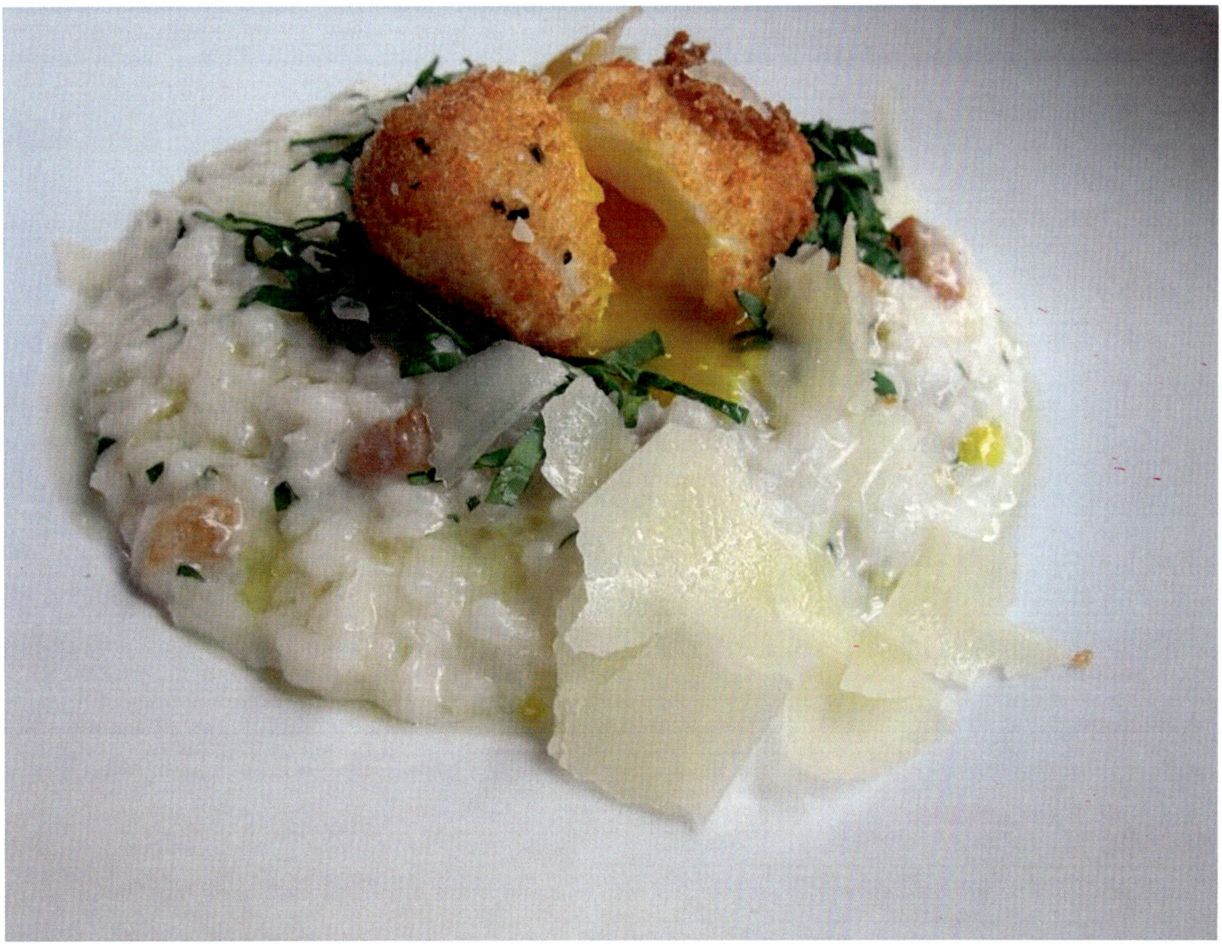

Prep Time: 10 minutes. Cook Time: 10 minutes. Total Time: 20 minutes.

Bacon and Egg Risotto is a great savory breakfast or brunch option. The best thing about this recipe, it's ready within just a few minutes!

Servings: 2

Ingredients

3 chopped slices center cut bacon
2 eggs
1½ cups chicken broth
¾ cup Arborio Rice
1/3 onions, chopped
3 tablespoons Dry White Wine
2 tablespoons Grated Parmesan Cheese
Chives, for garnish
Salt and Pepper, to taste

Instructions

1. Turn the Instant Pot on the "Sauté" function then add bacon. Cook for about 5 minutes until the fats start to render and the bacon is crisping.
2. Stir in the onion and let it cook for about 2-3 minutes.
3. Stir in the rice and let it sauté for a minute.
4. Pour in the wine and stir until the wine is absorbed, then add the chicken broth. Stir and cover the Instant Pot.
5. Set the valve to "Sealing" and change the setting to "Manual". Set the timer for 5 minutes.
6. Cook the eggs to your liking (poached, sunny side up, or over easy).
7. Quick Release the pressure and remove the lid once the rice is done cooking. Stir in the parmesan cheese, salt and pepper.
8. Serve in two plates, add the cooked egg and sprinkle the chives.
9. Enjoy!

Giant Instant Pot Pancake

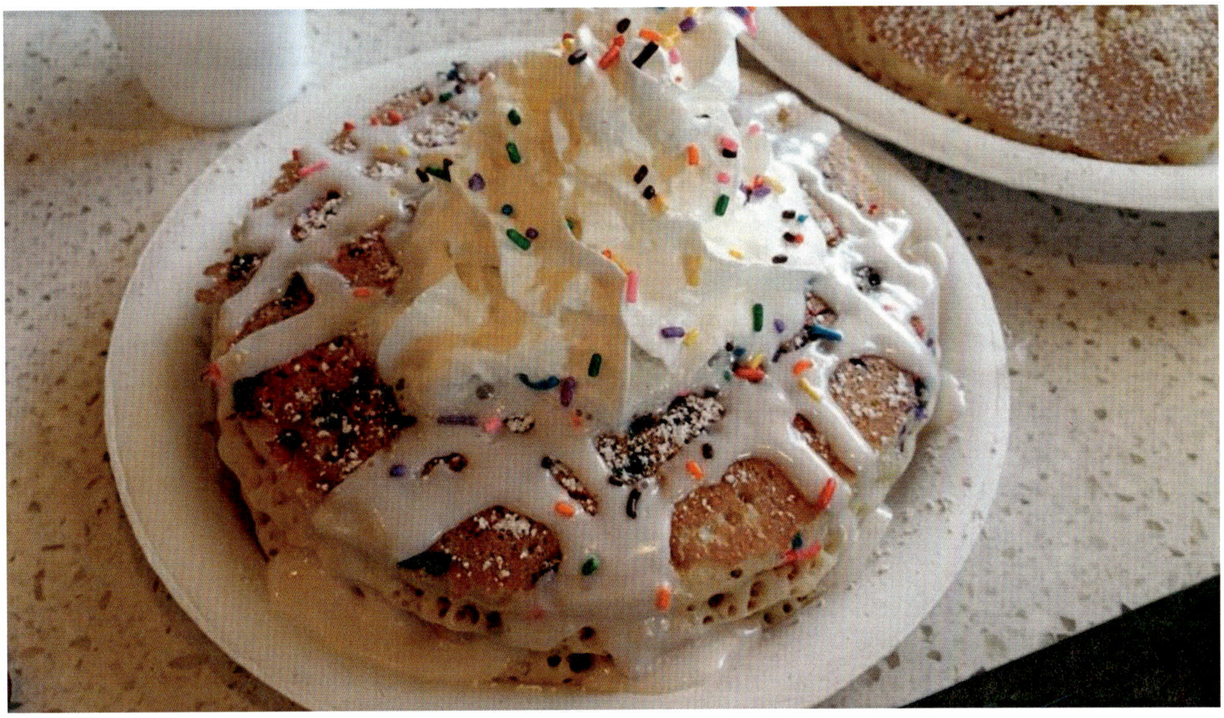

Prep Time: 5 minutes. Cook Time: 45 minutes. Total Time: 50 minutes.

The enormous Pancake is a thick and fluffy twist to the classic American breakfast pancakes. With a crispy top, the less chewy treat is perfect for any sweet tooth.

Servings: 6

Ingredients

2 cups all-purpose Flour
1½ cups Milk
2 large eggs
2 ½ tablespoons baking powder
2 tablespoons granulated white sugar

Instructions

1. Add the milk and eggs in a large mixing bowl and whisk them together. Add the remaining ingredients to the blended mixture and continue whisking until the batter is smooth.
2. Use a cooking spray to grease the interior of your inner pot. Then pour in the batter.
3. Seal the lid and ensure the vent is closed before programming your Instant Pot to the "Manual" function. Set the pressure to "Low Pressure" and set the cooking timer to 45 minutes.

4. Once the timer goes off, check whether your pancake is cooked. If the pancake isn't quite done yet, continue cooking it on low pressure for a few more seconds until its ready.
5. Use a spatula to loosen the cake from the sides of your inner pot and carefully pop the pancake out upside down. The top of your pancake should be crispy, golden brown.
6. Add your favorite pancake toppings and serve.
7. Enjoy!

Ham and Egg Casserole

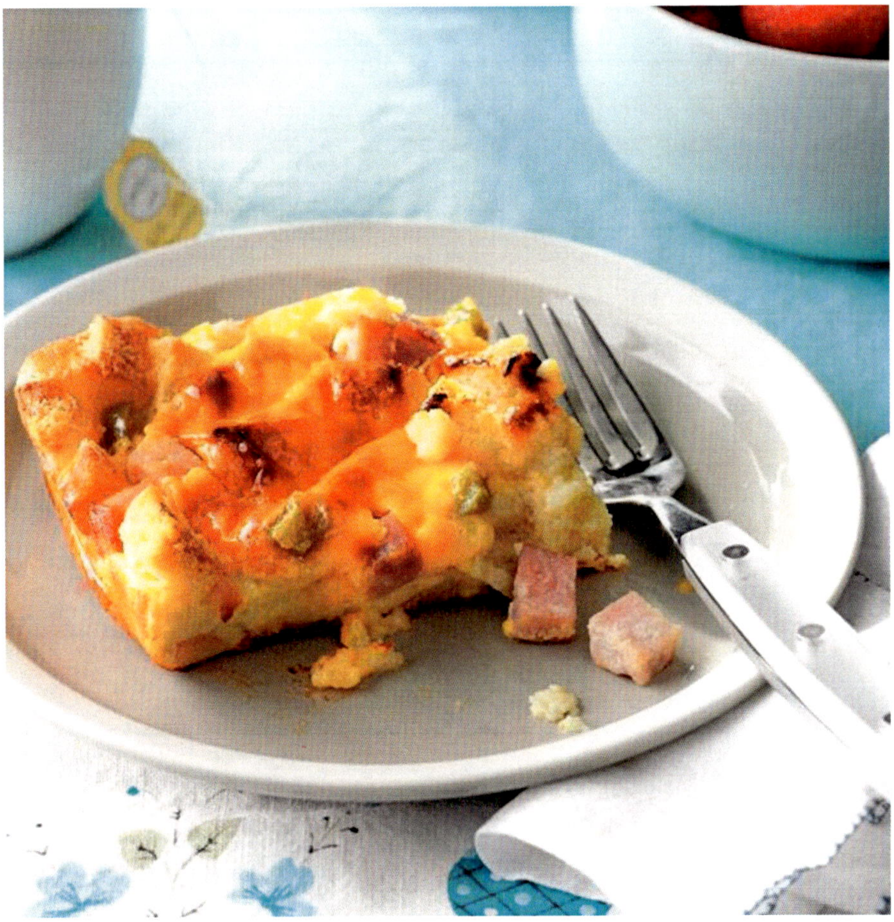

Prep Time: 5 minutes. Cook Time: 25 minutes. Total Time: 30 minutes.

If you like a delicious Egg Casserole for breakfast, this is a great easy-to-make recipe that actually works.

Servings: 4

Ingredients

4 medium red potatoes
10 large eggs
2 cups shredded cheddar cheese
1 cup chopped ham
1 cup milk
½ diced onion
1 teaspoon pepper
1 teaspoon salt

Toppings (Optional)

Salsa
Sour Cream

Avocado

Instructions

1. Grease the inner pot with non-stick cooking spray before adding milk and eggs. Whisk the mixture until it's well blended.
2. Place the potatoes, onions, ham, salt, and pepper in the blended mixture. Stir and cover the inner pot with foil.
3. Place the steam rack in the Instant Pot and add 2 cups of water.
4. Place the inner pot on the steam rack and seal the lid. Program your Instant Pot to "Manual" function and set the timer for 25 minutes.
5. Do a Quick Release when the timer goes off and unseal the lid immediately.
6. Add your favorite toppings and serve.
7. Enjoy!

Vanilla Latte Steel Cut Oats

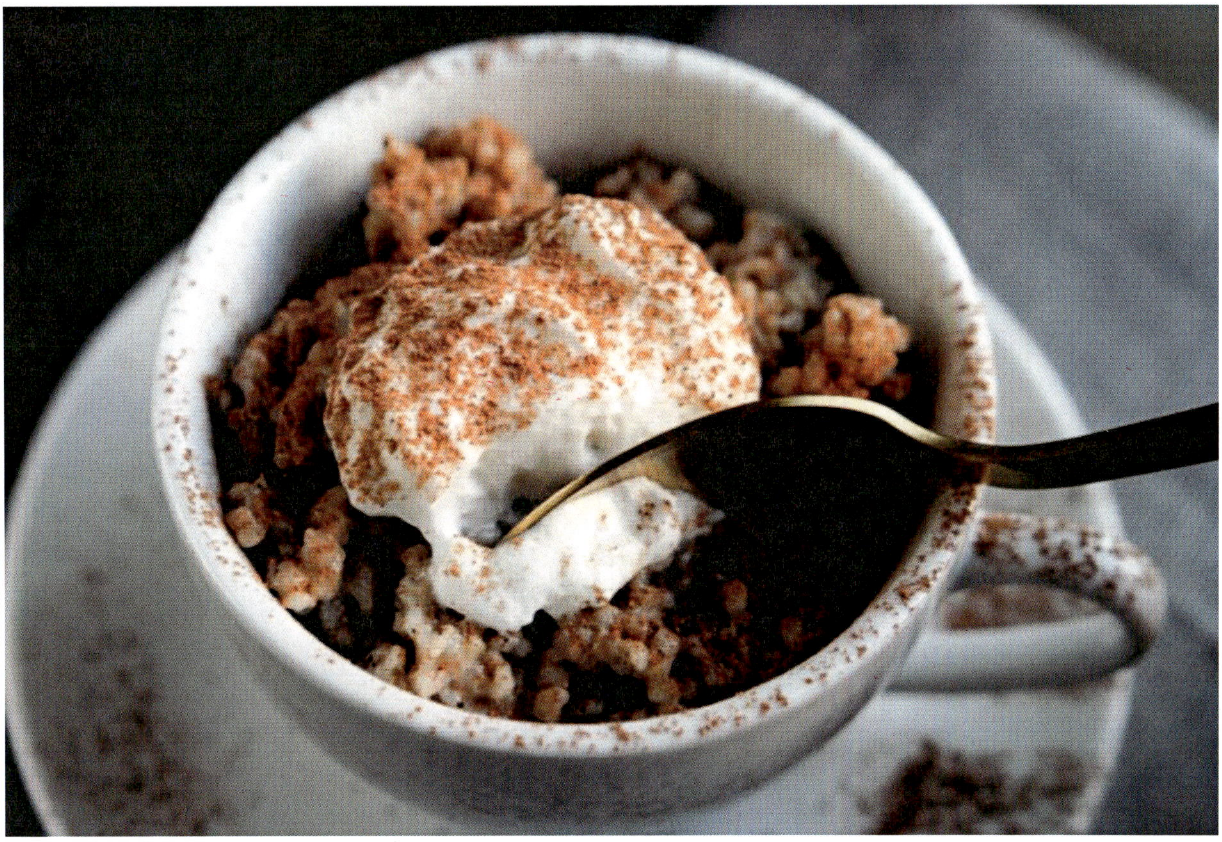

Prep Time: 10 minutes. Cook Time: 10 minutes. Total Time: 20 minutes.

This hearty breakfast gives you a caffeine kick by combining flavors from your daily coffee drink. The mild coffee flavor from the espresso powder is also perfect for kids, making Vanilla Steel Cut Oats a family breakfast treat. You can add more espresso powder for a stronger coffee flavor and chocolate syrup for your sweet tooth, either way, this is a delicious and healthy way to kick off your day.

Servings: 4

Ingredients

1 cup Steel Cut Oats
2 ½ cups water
1 cup milk
2 teaspoons vanilla extract
1 teaspoon espresso powder
2 tablespoons sugar
¼ teaspoon salt
Finely grates chocolate
Freshly whipped cream

Instructions

1. Add oats, milk, water, espresso powder, sugar, and salt to your inner pot and lower it into your Instant Pot. Stir the ingredients to dissolve the espresso powder.
2. Seal the lid. Select the "High Pressure" function and set the cook time to 10 minutes.
3. Allow Natural Pressure Release for 10 minutes after the timer goes off. Then do Quick Pressure Release before carefully removing the lid.
4. Stir in additional sugar and vanilla extract to taste. Cover the lid and let the oats sit for 5 minutes until they get to your desired thickness.
5. Serve topped with finely grated chocolate and freshly whipped cream.
6. Enjoy!

Banana French Toast

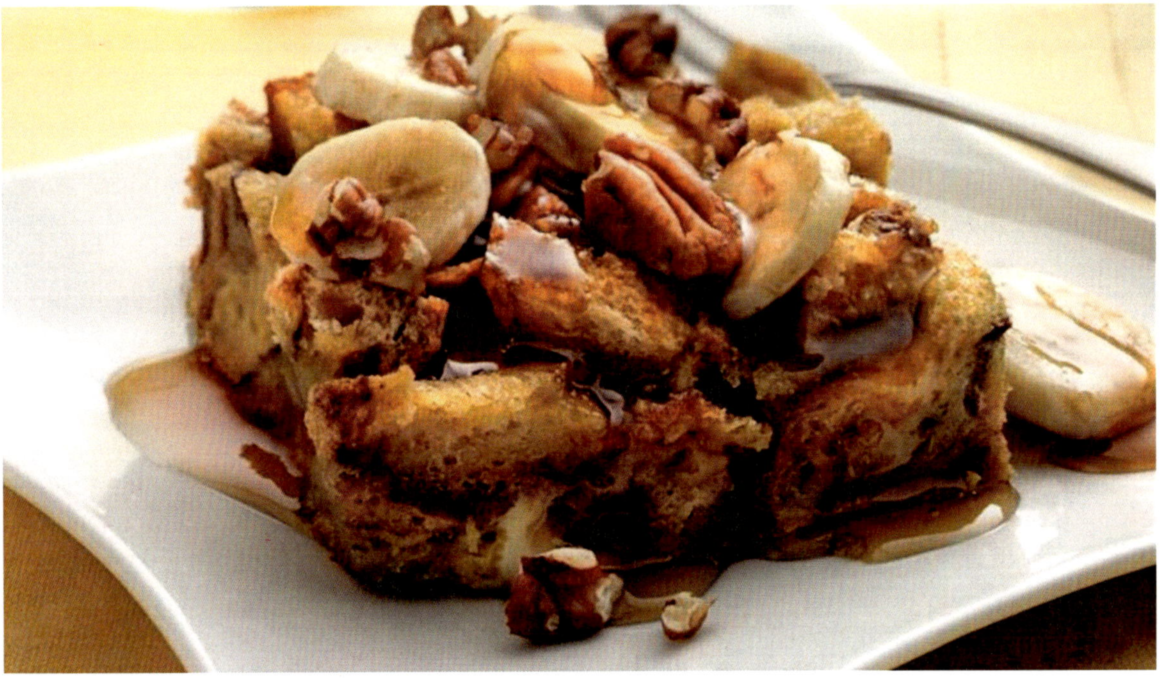

Prep Time: 15 minutes. Cook Time: 5 minutes. Total Time: 20 minutes.

Everybody likes French Toast. This easy Banana French Toast recipe is great for a quick breakfast meal or even brunch. Topped with maple syrup, nuts, and bananas this recipe might end up being your go-to breakfast meal. No worries if you not like banana, leave them out the recipe will still taste as good.

Servings: 6.

Ingredients

4 bananas, thinly sliced
6 slices French bread, cut into ¾ inch cubes
¼ cup milk
¼ cup cream cheese
¼ cup pecans, chopped
3 eggs
2 tablespoons butter
2 tablespoons brown sugar
1 tablespoon white sugar
1 teaspoon vanilla extract
½ teaspoon ground cinnamon

Optional

Maple syrup

Instructions

1. Generously grease a round baking dish or a cake pan that fits inside your Instant Pot.
2. Place a layer of bread on the greased baking dish and add a layer of one sliced banana on top of the bread. Sprinkle a tablespoon of brown sugar over the bananas.
3. Melt the cream cheese in the microwave and spread over the bread and banana layers. Add the remaining bread to the dish and add another layer of sliced banana. Sprinkle the remaining tablespoon of brown sugar over the sliced banana top with half the pecans. Slice the butter and place it as the top layer.
4. Beat eggs in a mixing bowl and whisk in the milk, vanilla, white sugar and cinnamon. Pour the egg mixture into the baking dish and ensure that you coat the bread well.
5. Pour ¾ cup water into the Instant Pot and place a steam rack trivet into the pot. Place the baking dish on the trivet and close the lid
6. Program the Instant Pot to "Porridge" setting then set cook time to 5 minutes. Once the timer goes off do a Quick Pressure Release. Leave the lid on for another 5 minutes and carefully remove the lid and the dish.
7. Serve topped with sliced bananas, maple syrup, and nuts.
8. Enjoy!

Apple-Squash Porridge

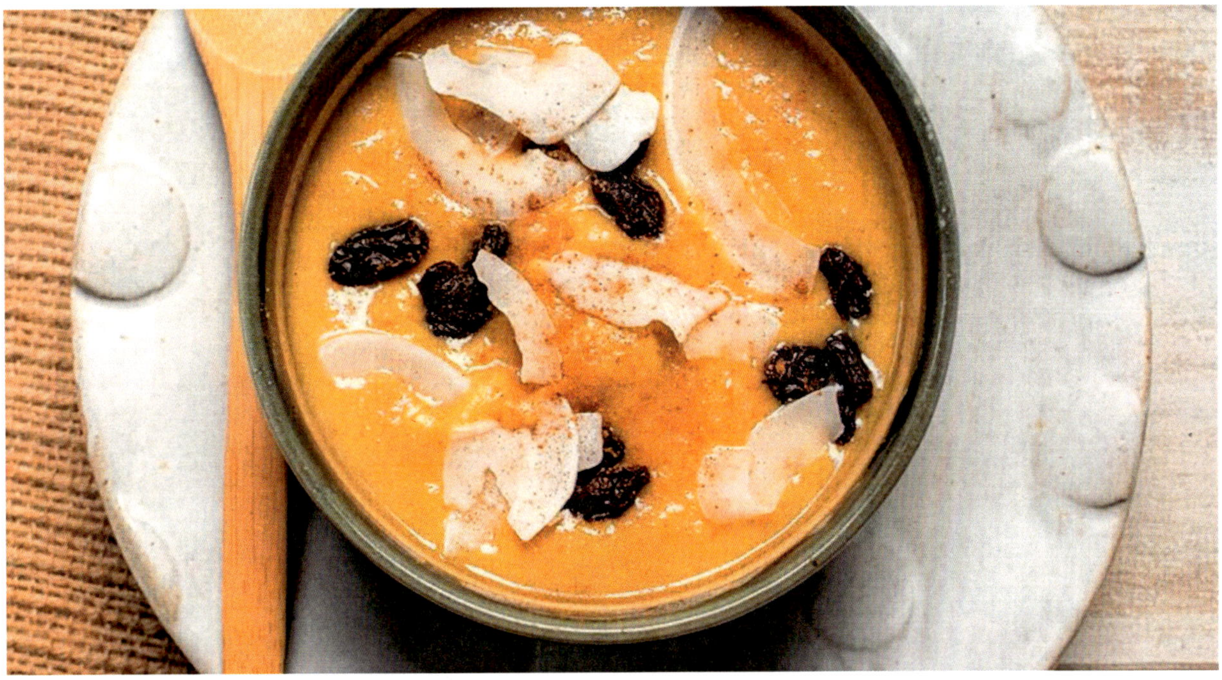

Prep Time: 10 minutes. Cook Time: 10 minutes. Total Time: 20 minutes.

Enjoy Apple-Squash Porridge hot for breakfast or chill it and enjoy as a pudding. The wholesome porridge recipe is great for the family, and the kids will love it. Apple-Squash Porridge is delicious and naturally sweet.

Servings: 3

Ingredients

2 large or 4 small apples, cut into chunks
1 whole Delicata squash
¼ cup gelatin
½ cup water or bone broth
2 tablespoon maple syrup
3 tablespoons slippery elm
½ teaspoon cinnamon
1/8 teaspoon ginger
1/8 teaspoon cloves
1 pinch salt

Instructions

1. Place the whole Delicata squash in the inner pot, pour the bone broth then add apple chunks and spices. Close the lid and ensure the Pressure Release Valve is set to "Sealing" position.
2. Program the Instant Pot to "Manual" setting and set the cook time to 8 minutes.

3. Allow Natural Pressure Release for about 10 minutes after the timer goes off. Carefully open the lid and set the pot's contents aside to cool.
4. Cut the cooled squash to half length-wise. Use a spoon to remove the seeds. Place the squash and all the other pot's content in a blender.
5. Blend the mixture to a puree then add a pinch of salt, maple syrup, slippery elm and gelatin and continue blending for an additional 30 seconds.
6. Serve with your favorite toppings and enjoy!

Breakfast Burrito Casserole

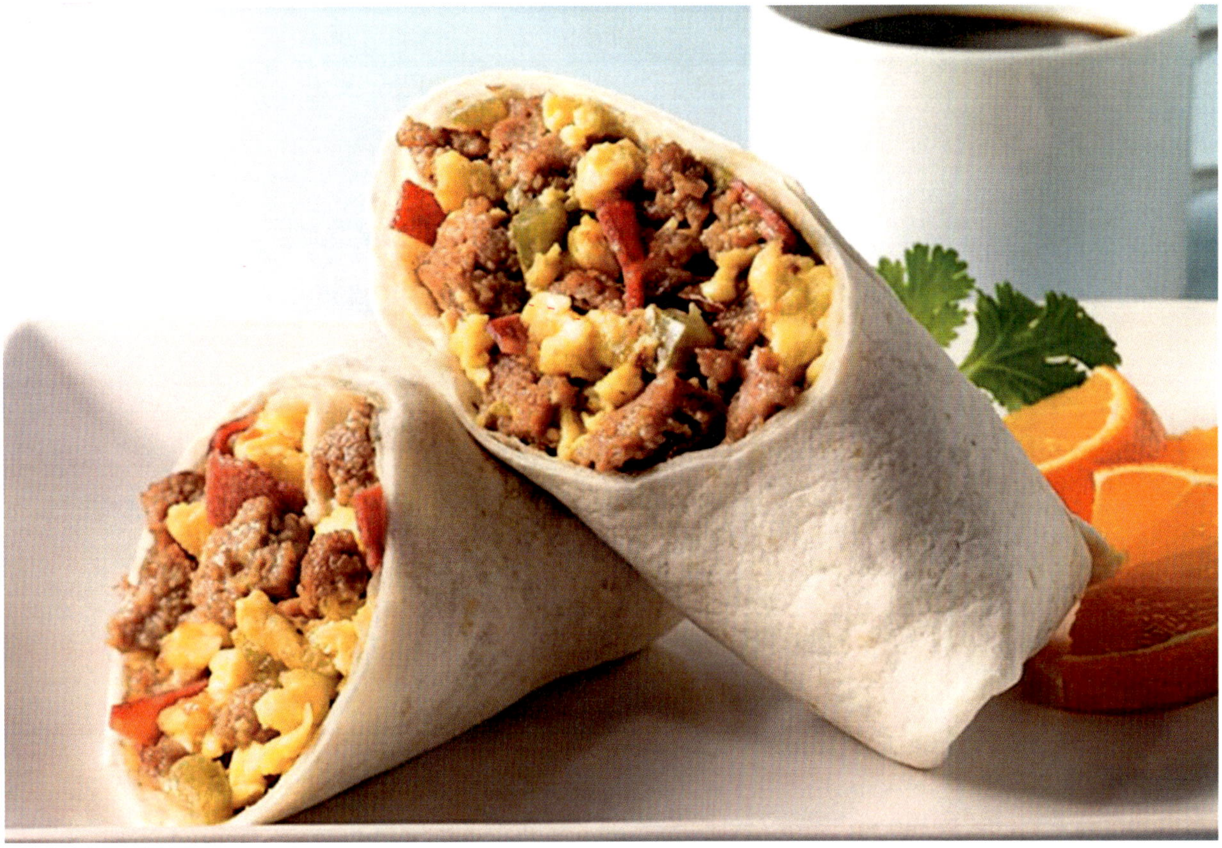

Prep Time: 10 minutes. Cook Time: 13 minutes. Total Time: 23 minutes.

Breakfast has never been this easy. The Instant Pot Breakfast Burrito Casserole recipe attests to easy cooking. All you have to do is chop stuff up, and your breakfast is ready in no time. All the ingredients are available in your kitchen.

Servings: 6.

Ingredients

2 lbs red potatoes, cubed
4 eggs
6 oz ham steak, cubed
¼ cup yellow or white onion, chopped
1 jalapeno, diced
¾ teaspoon taco seasoning
½ teaspoon mesquite seasoning
¼ teaspoon chili powder
½ teaspoon salt
Tortillas

Burrito toppings

Marinated red onions
Salsa
Hot sauce
Avocado

Instructions

1. In a medium bowl beat the eggs and whisk in salt, seasonings and a tablespoon of water. Then add onions, jalapeno, potatoes and ham into the bowl.
2. Pour this mixture into an inner pot and cover with a lid or foil.
3. Add 1 cup of water into the Instant Pot then place the trivet into the Pot. Place the bowl with the egg mixture on the trivet then close the Instant Pot lid.
4. Ensure the Pressure Release Vent is set to "Sealing" position. Program the Instant Pot to "Manual" and cook at "High Pressure" for 13 minutes.
5. Allow Natural Pressure Release once the timer goes off. Carefully open the lid and remove the inner pot.

Fill the burritos

6. Heat up each side of the tortilla in a skillet. Add a few scoops of the egg mixture, red onions, salsa, avocado and hot sauce (if desired) in each burrito. Refrigerate leftover filling in an airtight container for later.
7. Wrap up, serve and enjoy!

Yogurt with Fruit

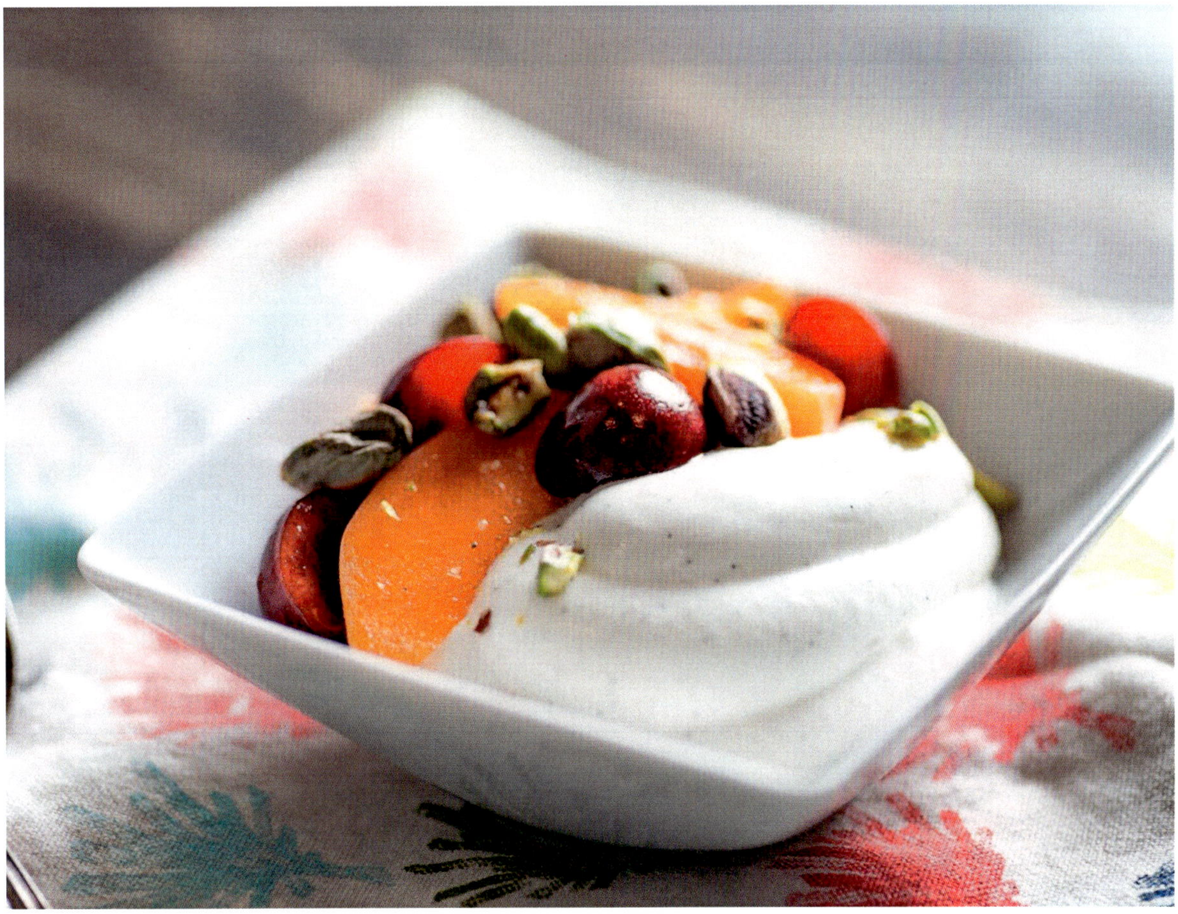

Prep Time: 5 minutes. Cook Time: 9 hours. Total Time: 9 hours 05 minutes.

This Instant Pot Yogurt with Fruit recipe makes a delicious and healthier homemade Yogurt drink. Yogurt with Fruit makes a great breakfast and kids love it. The homemade Yogurt comes in handy as a quick grab-and-go breakfast on those late mornings.

Servings: 4-6

Ingredients

½ cup Greek Yogurt
1 gallon milk, divided (½ gallon whole, ½ gallon 2%)
2 cups fruit
1 cup sugar
2 tablespoons vanilla bean paste

Instructions

1. Pour the milk into the Inner Pot and place it in the Instant Pot. Seal the lid. Program the Instant Pot to "Yogurt" function. Press the "Adjust" button until it gets to "Boil" setting and cook for about 45 minutes.

2. Once the timer goes off, carefully open the lid and set aside the milk to cool to about 115F.
3. Place the milk back into the Instant Pot. Use a wooden spoon to whisk in ½ cup of Greek Yogurt then add 2 tablespoons of vanilla bean paste.
4. Set the Instant Pot to "Yogurt" function and allow the Instant Pot to count up from 0:00 to 8 hours.
5. Once the Yogurt is ready, use cloth napkins or nut milk bags to strain it. Store the Yogurt in glass jars and chill in the refrigerator.
6. Boil 1 cup sugar, and 2 cups fruits then set aside to cool.
7. In small containers divide the fruit mixture and top up with Yogurt.
8. Serve and enjoy!

Egg Brûlée

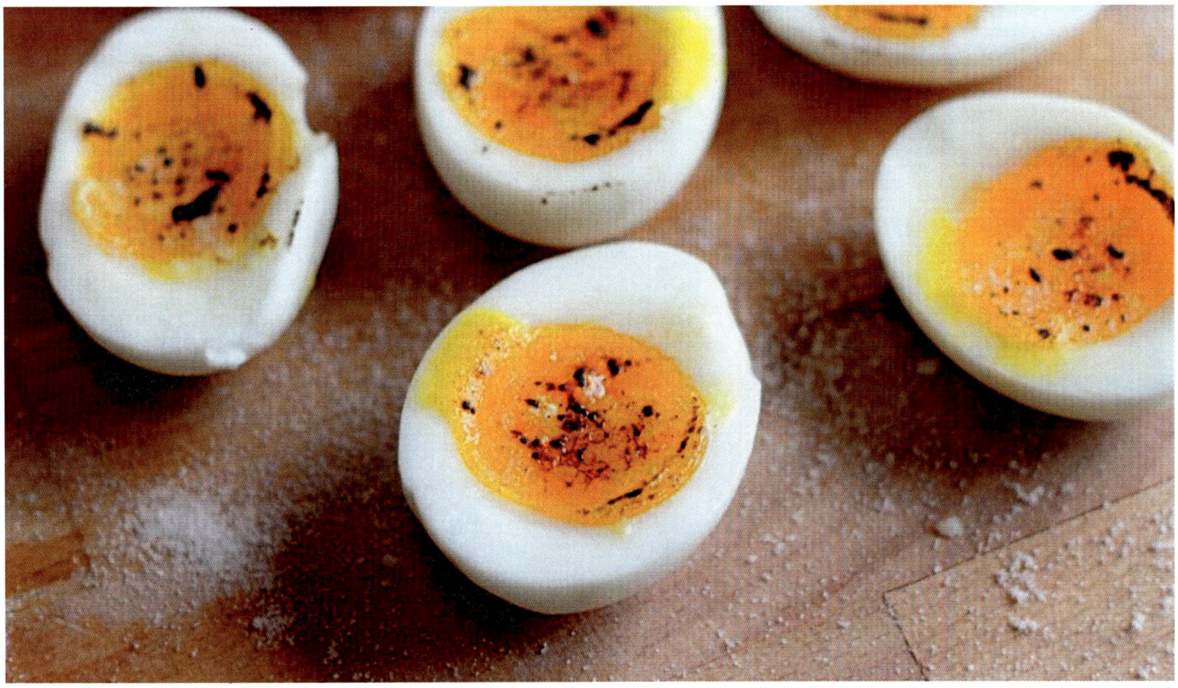

Prep Time: 5 minutes. Cook Time: 3 minutes. Total Time: 8 minutes.

It's always a somewhat tricky task to cook eggs in the Instant Pot, something that makes this recipe an even trickier and fun task to undertake. The 3-ingredient recipe presents an opportunity to impress your family or guests with a fancy yet so simple appetizer. Egg Brûlée makes a yummy treat for parties and potlucks.

Servings: 6

Ingredients

6 large eggs
1 cup water
Granulated sugar and table salt to taste

Instructions

1. Pour 1 cup of water into the Instant Pot and place a trivet in the pot. Place the eggs on the trivet and seal the lid.
2. Program the Instant Pot to "High Pressure" and cook for 3 minutes. Once the timer goes off, do a Quick Release.
3. Careful open the lid and cool the eggs in a cold-water bath.
4. Peel the eggs gently under running tap water. Using a paring knife cut the eggs in half lengthwise. Sprinkle a pinch of granulated sugar and a pinch of salt over the halved eggs.
5. Using a culinary torch caramelize the sugar to until it forms a crispy top.
6. Serve and enjoy!

APPETIZERS AND SIDES

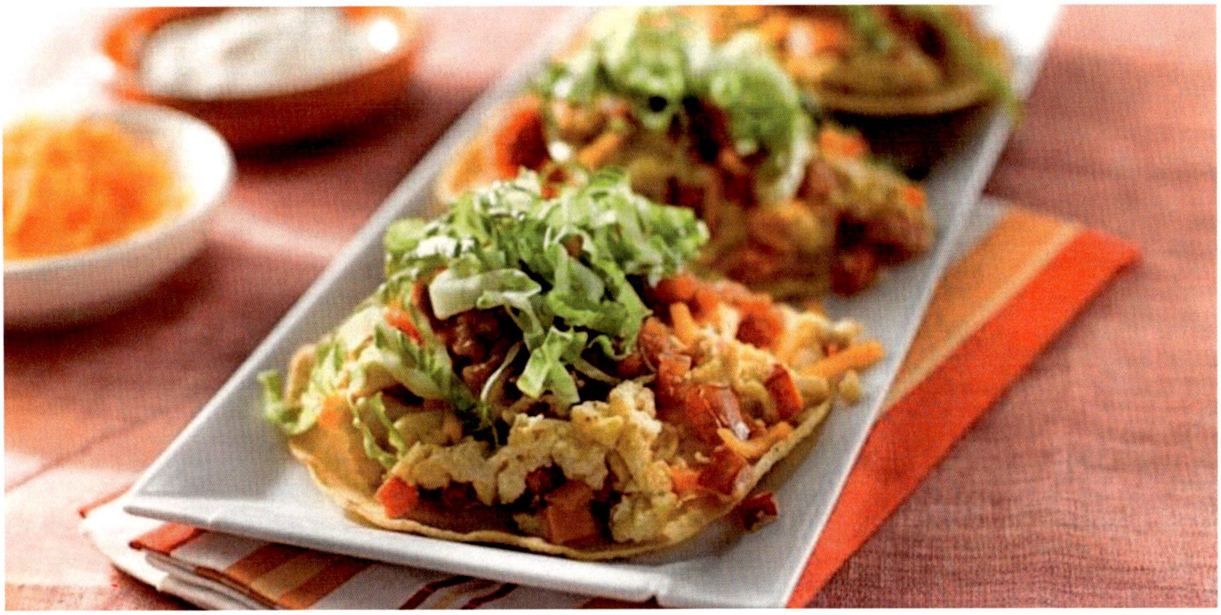

Appetizers and sides are a perfect way of completing a feast, meal or even keep your guests entertained during a party. With an Instant Pot, you can make unlimited appetizers and delicious dishes for your family and guests. Spice up main dishes by pairing them up with any of the creative or classic side dishes below. Almost all the Instant Pot appetizers and sides are easy to make, deliciously yummy and perfect whether your dinner is creative or traditional. There are endless possibilities for an amazing and unforgettable meal with these healthy appetizers and side dishes.

Buffalo Chicken Meatballs

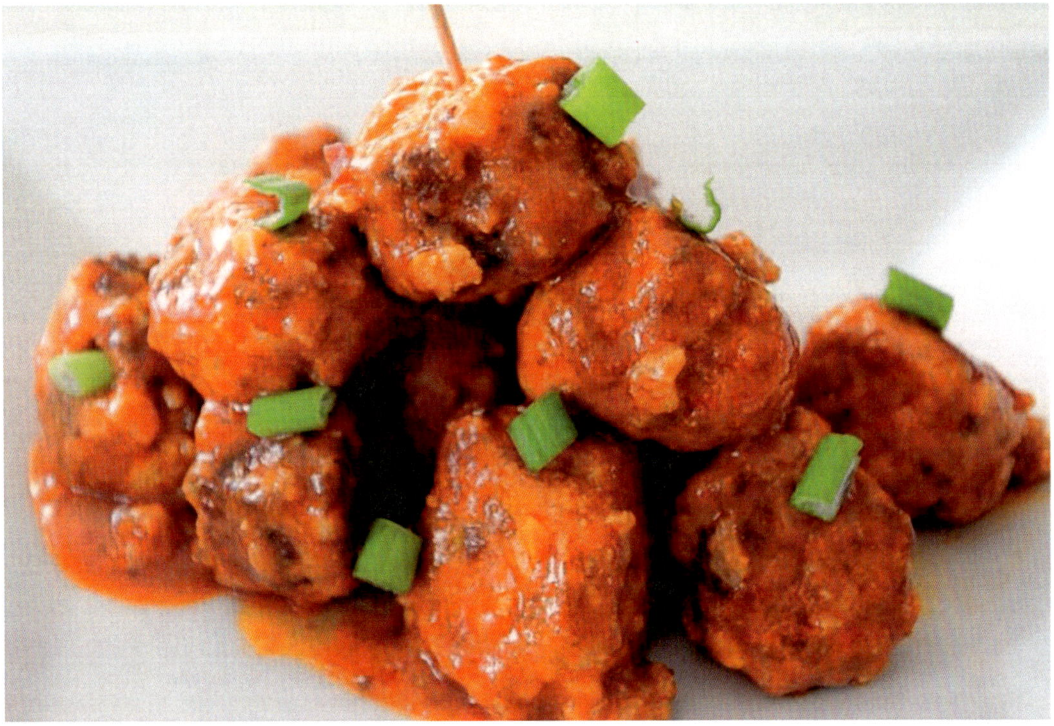

Prep Time: 10 minutes. Cook Time: 20 minutes. Total Time: 30 minutes.

It's no question that buffalo sauce flavored dishes are a favorite in most households and even more popular during sporting events and gatherings. The spicy kick of Instant Pot Buffalo Chicken Meatballs is yummy and addictive. The dish has tasty delicious flavors, and it's less messy because you don't have to deal with bones. Don't worry if the meatballs don't perfectly take shape immediately; they'll firm up once they are ready.

Servings: 6

Ingredients

1.5 lbs ground chicken
2 green onions, thinly sliced
2 garlic cloves, minced
¾ cup almond meal
6 tablespoons hot sauce
4 tablespoons ghee or butter
2 tablespoons ghee
1 teaspoon sea salt

Optional

Green onions, chopped. For garnish.

Instructions

Chicken meatballs

1. Add the chicken, green onions, almond meal, minced garlic and salt into a large bowl. Use both hands to carefully mix the ingredients without overworking the meat.
2. Use coconut oil or ghee to grease your hands before shaping the meat into medium balls (about 1-2 inches wide).
3. Program your Instant Pot to "Sauté" function and add 2 tablespoons of ghee.
4. Working in batches, brown the chicken meatballs in the Instant Pot. Turn them periodically until all the sides are brown.

Buffalo sauce

5. As the meatballs are browning in the Instant Pot, combine the 4 tablespoons of ghee or butter and the hot sauce. Heat the combination until the butter melts completely.
6. Use a spoon to stir the ingredients.

Buffalo chicken meatballs

7. Place all your browned meatballs in the Instant Pot and evenly pour in the buffalo sauce.
8. Seal the lid and set the pressure valve to "sealing."
9. Program the Instant Pot to "Poultry" function and set the timer for 10 minutes.
10. Once the timer goes off, release the pressure valve or let Instant Pot automatically switch to "Keep Warm" mode.
11. You can eat the Buffalo chicken wings as a single dish, or you could serve them over noodles, rice or cauliflower rice.
12. Enjoy!

Spinach Artichoke Dip

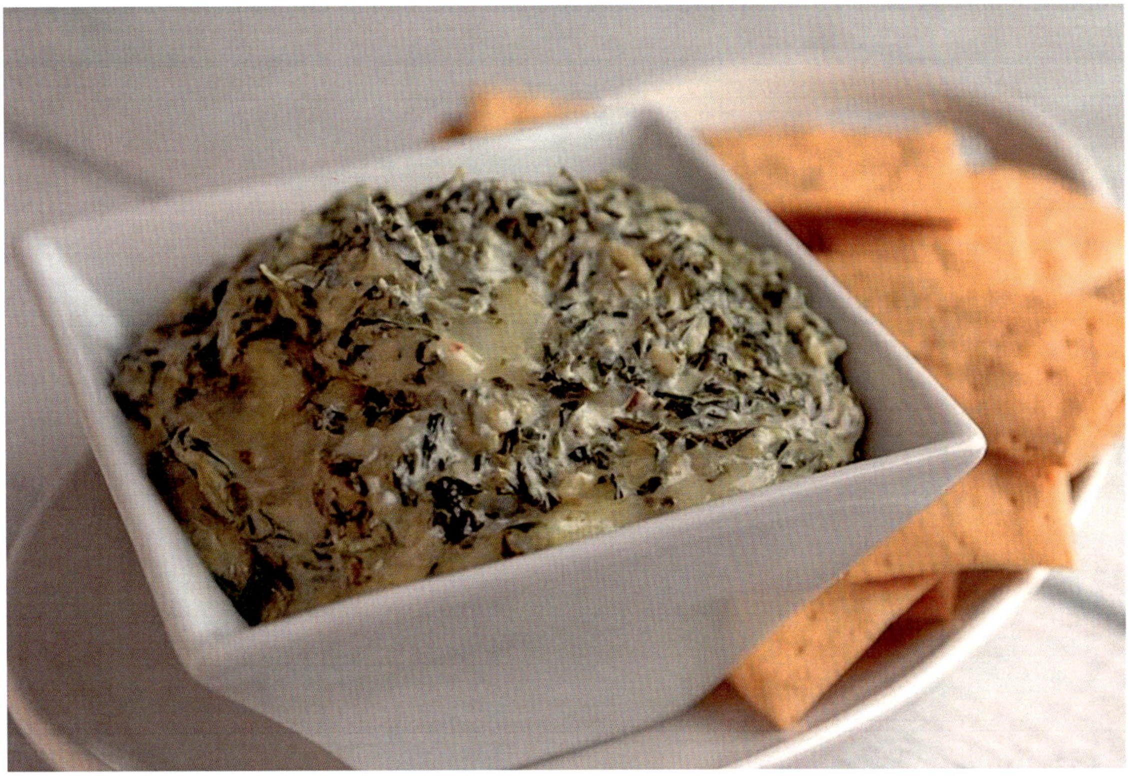

Prep Time: 10 minutes. Cook Time: 10 minutes. Total Time: 20 minutes.

Spinach Artichoke dip is a 10-minute easy-to-make tasty Instant Pot recipe when you need a simple and healthy appetizer. For a brown top on your dip, sprinkle the cheese and leave the dish in the oven for a few minutes.

Servings: 6

Ingredients

1 box frozen spinach, chopped
1 can artichoke hearts, drained and chopped
1 block cream cheese
½ cup onions, finely chopped
2 cloves garlic, minced
1 cup shredded mozzarella cheese
½ grated parmesan cheese
½ cup Greek Yogurt
1 teaspoon Worcestershire sauce
Salt and pepper to taste

Instructions

1. Defrost the spinach for 1 minute in the microwave, then add all ingredients to a mixing bowl.

2. Stir the ingredients and transfer the mixture to an oven-safe baking dish and cover it with foil.
3. Add 1 cup of water into the Instant Pot and place the steam rack. Then lower the dish in your Instant Pot.
4. Seal the lid and set the Instant Pot to "High Pressure" setting then set the time for 10 minutes.
5. Set the steam release valve to "Venting" once the timer goes off, to release the pressure. Carefully remove the dish after the all the pressure is released and remove the foil.
6. Serve your Spinach Artichoke Dip hot with crackers, tortilla chips or a sliced baguette.
7. Enjoy!

Instant Pot Hummus

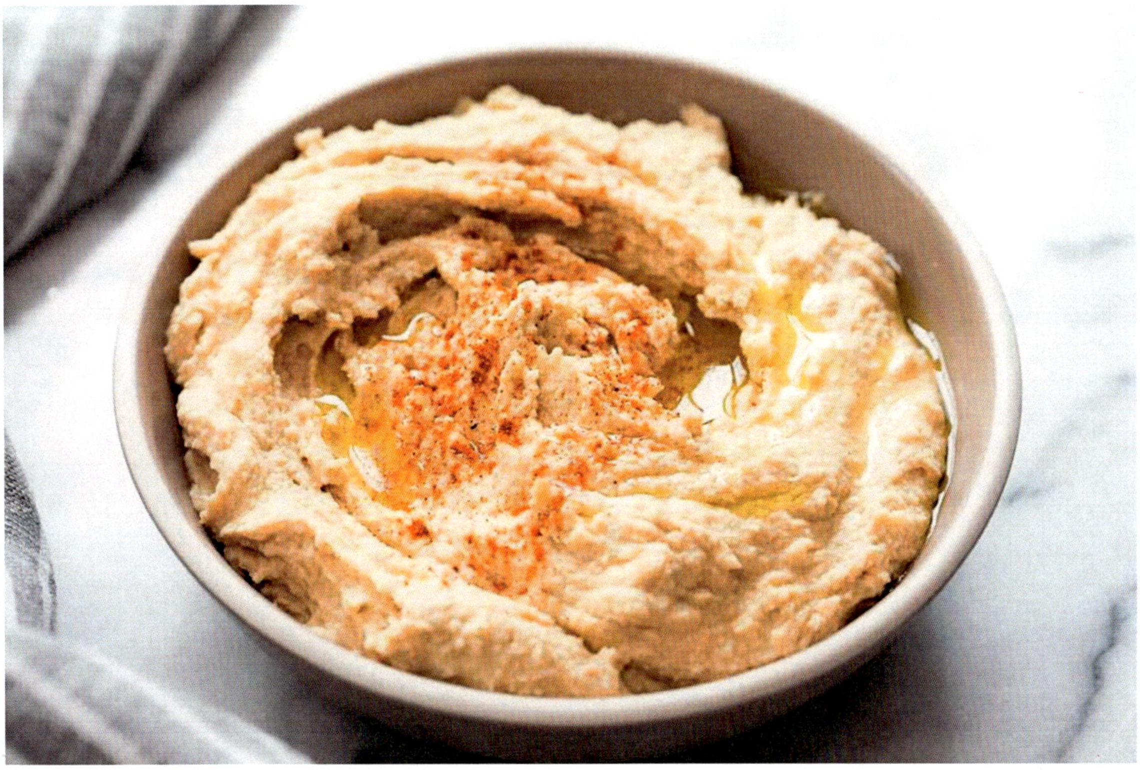

Prep Time: 20 minutes. Cook Time: 45 minutes. Total Time:1 hour 05 minutes.

You can easily make your own Hummus from scratch using simple ingredients such as garlic, lemon juice and olive oil that are readily available in your kitchen. Hummus is a healthy and creamy dip that goes perfectly well with raw veggies and crackers. You can also serve kids the hummus with baby carrots, celery sticks, pita or wheat thins. For this recipe, you don't need tahini, but it tastes just as great if not better with the tahini.

Servings: 10

Ingredients

¾ cup dried chickpeas
3 cups water
1 garlic clove, minced
1 tablespoon lemon juice, fresh
2 tablespoons olive oil
1 tablespoon salt

Optional

Parsley
Red pepper flakes
Freshly ground pepper

Instructions

1. Add water, salt and the chickpeas to the Instant Pot and seal the lid. Ensure the valve is set to "Sealing."
2. Program the Instant Pot to "Manual" setting and set the timer for 45 minutes.
3. Move the valve to "Venting" once the timer goes off and let the pot sit for 5 minutes.
4. Use a strainer or sieve to drain the liquid from the chickpeas. Reserve the drained liquid for later.
5. Add ¼ cup of the reserved liquid, lemon juice, olive oil, garlic and lastly the chickpeas in a blender or food processor. Blend until the mixture is thick and creamy (you can always add more of the reserved liquid to your desired consistency).
6. Season to taste and add the optional toppings as you desire.
7. Immediately serve or store the hummus in an airtight container in the refrigerator for later (up to a week).
8. Enjoy!

Chicken Tikka Bites

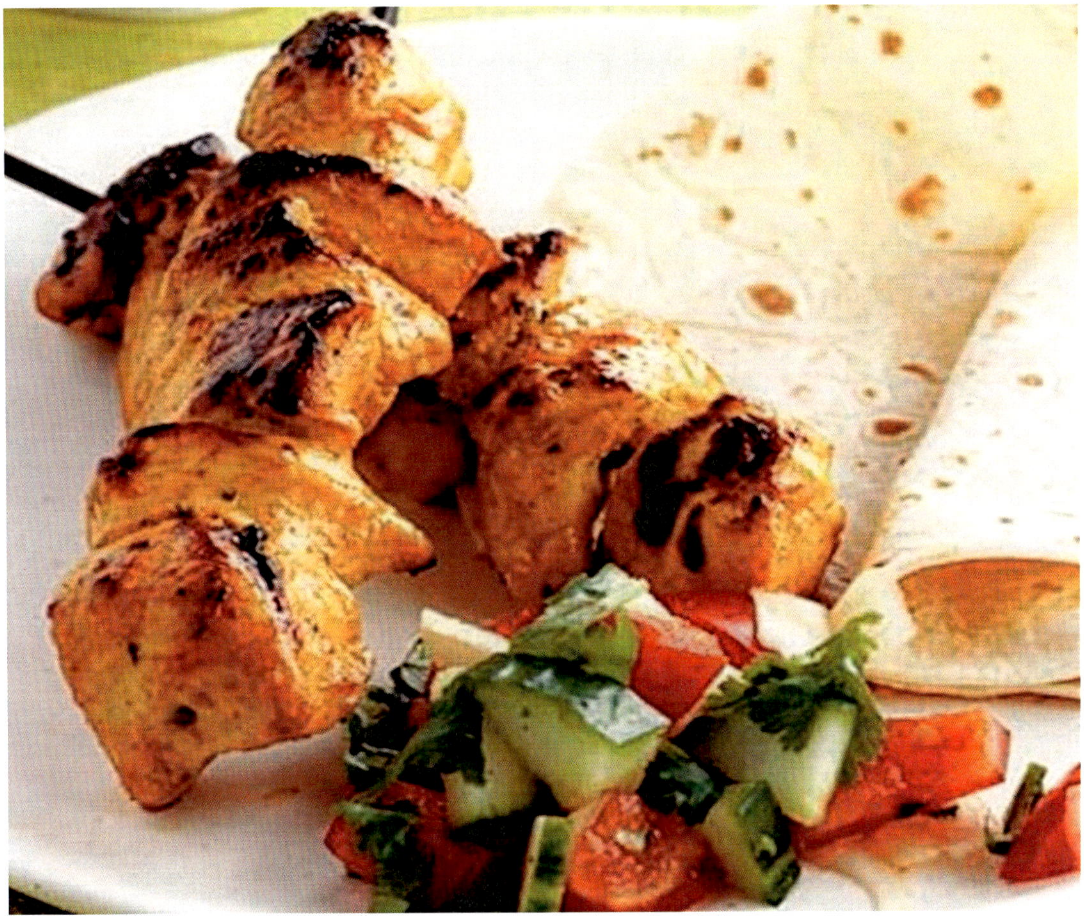

Prep Time: 2 hours 03 minutes. Cook Time: 4 minutes. Total Time: 2 hours 07 minutes.

Chicken Tikka Bites are perfect served hot or cold. It's an easy-to-cook Instant Pot recipe without any wash-up, making it the perfect meal. This recipe is based on a single serving, but you can double or triple the ingredients to add the yield.

Servings: 1

Ingredients

- 1 chicken breast
- ½ lemon and rind
- 3 tablespoons Greek Yogurt
- 1 tablespoon mixed spice
- 1 tablespoon masala powder
- 1 tablespoon garam masala
- 1 tablespoon turmeric
- 1 tablespoon cumin
- 1 tablespoon coriander
- 1 tablespoon chili powder
- 1 tablespoon garlic puree

1 tablespoon ginger puree
Salt and pepper to taste.

Instructions

1. Place all the seasoning onto a foil. Season the chicken breast with salt and pepper and place it on the foil.
2. Add the Greek Yogurt and drizzle the lemon juice on the chicken breast.
3. Seal the foil and use a rolling pin to bash the ingredients in the foil. This allows the flavoring to spread.
4. Then transfer the sealed foil to the fridge and let it marinate for a couple of hours.
5. Add 1 cup of water into the Instant Pot and place the steam rack. Place the foil packet on the steam rack.
6. Seal the lid and set the valve to "Sealing." Program the Instant Pot to the "Steam" function and set the timer for 4 minutes.
7. Allow the Instant Pot to switch to "Keep Warm" function for a few minutes after the timer goes off before serving.
8. Slice the chicken breast to chunks and serve on a skewer or with a salad.
9. Enjoy!

Potato Salad

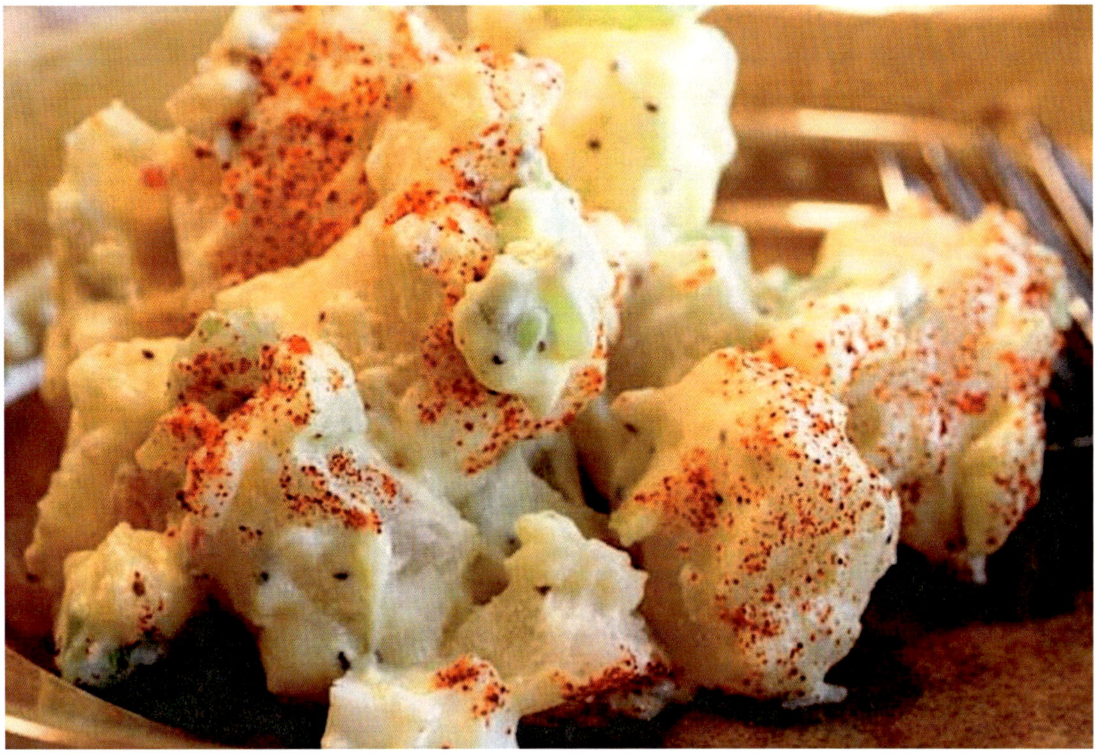

Prep Time: 15 minutes. Cook Time: 30 minutes. Total Time: 45 minutes.

Potato salad might be one of the easiest classic sides that most people make, however, a perfect potato salad is almost impossible to come by. Make a crunchy, creamy and fluffy potato salad in the Instant Pot. The salad dressing is rich, flavorful and light balancing the sweet, savory and tangy flavors. Get to enjoy the wholesome textures and flavors of the potato salad and the best part is you get to cook the egg and potatoes at the same time with no bowl or extra rack.

Servings: 8-12

Ingredients

3 1/3 lbs russet potatoes, peeled and cut into 1-inch cubes
4 cups water
3 tablespoons apple cider vinegar or unseasoned rice vinegar
2 ½ teaspoons fine table salt

Dressing

3 large eggs
1 cup full-fat mayonnaise
1 cornichon or dill pickle, diced
8-10 stems fresh dill, finely chopped
3 celery stalks, finely chopped
1 small red onion, finely diced
1 tablespoon apple cider vinegar or unseasoned rice vinegar

1 tablespoon whole grain mustard
½ teaspoon garlic powder
Black pepper and kosher salt to taste

Instructions

1. Add 4 cups of water, I tablespoon of apple cider vinegar or unseasoned rice vinegar and 2 ½ tablespoons of fine table salt in the Instant Pot. Layer the 3 eggs on top of the potatoes.
2. Seal the lid set the Instant Pot to "Low Pressure" and "Venting" the cook time will be approximately 23-24 minutes.
3. Once the timer goes off release the pressure immediately before carefully opening the lid.
4. Place the hard-boiled eggs in cold water. Let the potatoes cubes sit longer in hot water if they are not done then drain them with a colander.
5. Layer the hot potatoes on a large tray for them to cool. Drizzle 2 tablespoons of apple cider vinegar or unseasoned rice vinegar on the hot potato cube.
6. Once the hard-boiled eggs have cooled, chop them into small pieces.

Salad dressing

7. Add the finely diced and chopped ingredients, 1 cup mayonnaise, 1 tablespoon apple cider vinegar or unseasoned rice vinegar, 1 tablespoon whole grain mustard, ½ tablespoon garlic powder and finely chopped hard-boiled egg into a large mixing bowl.
8. Use a spatula to mix the ingredients. Drizzle in the fresh dill and continue mixing the ingredients.
9. Add the already cool potatoes into the mixing bowl and gently fold them into the combination using the spatula. Be careful not to overmix the potato salad. Add freshly ground black pepper and kosher salt to your desired taste.
10. Cover the potato salad and refrigerate for at least 3 hours.
11. Serve as a side dish and enjoy!

Instant Pot Salsa

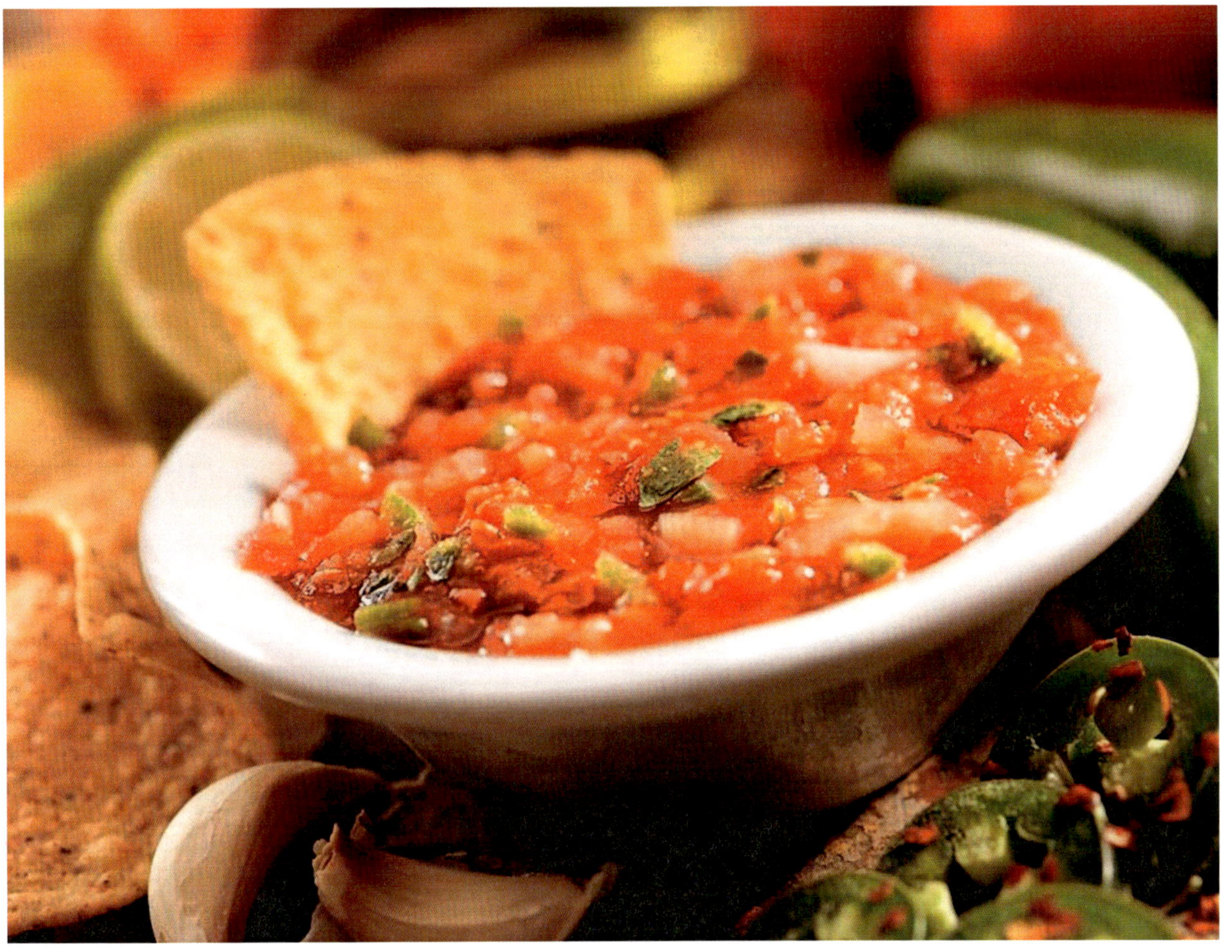

Prep Time: 10 minutes. Cook Time: 30 minutes. Total Time: 40 minutes.

Instant Pot Salsa is an easy-to-make and freezer friendly appetizer. The amazing thing about this recipe is that you can quickly prepare it and have it ready from your freezer whenever you need it.

Servings: 6-8

Ingredients

12 cups fresh tomatoes, peeled, seeded and diced
3 cans tomato paste
3 large yellow onions, diced
2 medium green peppers, diced
1 cup jalapeno pepper, seeded and chopped
½ cup vinegar
3 tablespoons cayenne pepper
3 tablespoons sugar
2 tablespoons garlic powder
1 tablespoon salt

Optional

4 tablespoons cilantro

Instructions

1. Add all the ingredients in the Instant Pot and stir the mixture
2. Seal the lid and set the Instant Pot to "Manual" function and set the timer for 30 minutes on "High Pressure."
3. Once the timer goes off, allow Natural Pressure Release and carefully open the lid.
4. Once the salsa cools can it and store in the refrigerator or freeze in airtight containers.

Black Bean Dip

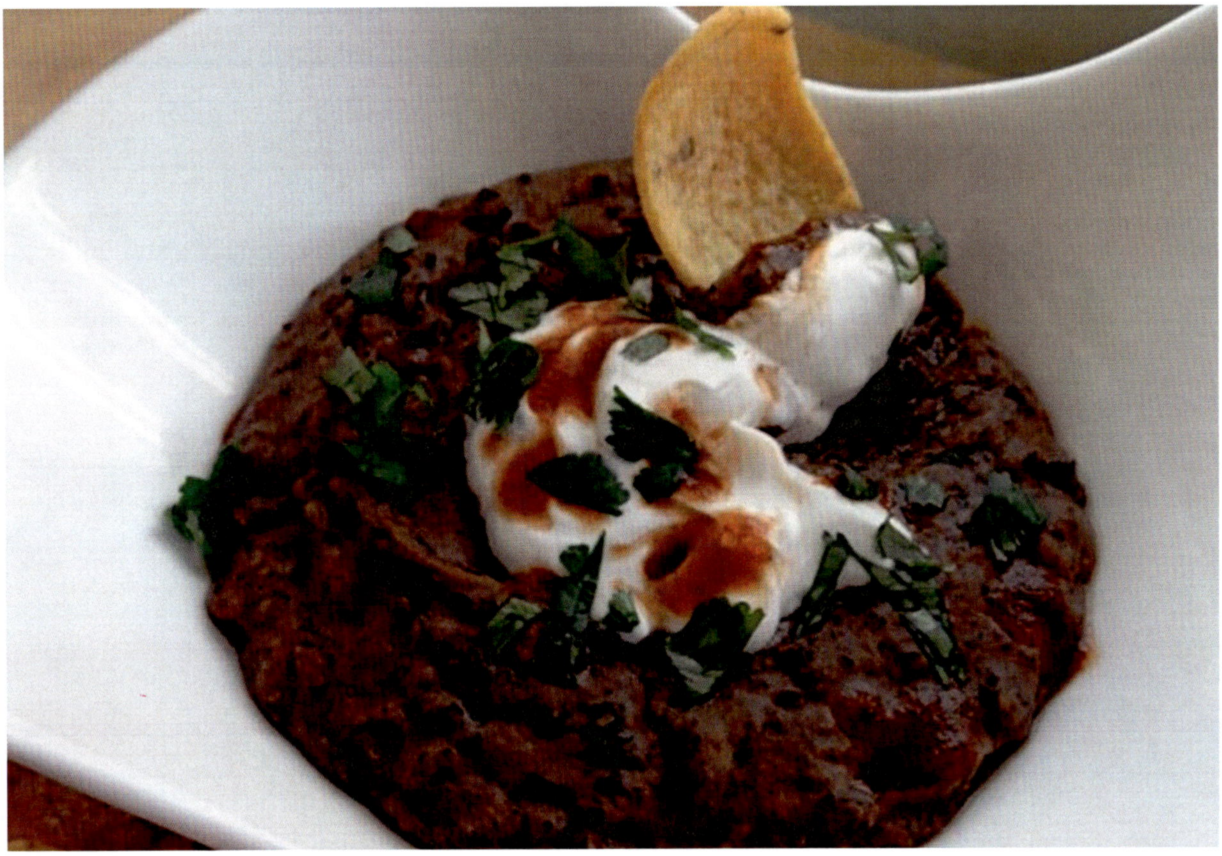

Prep Time: 15 minutes. Cook Time: 30 minutes. Total Time: 45 minutes.

This make-ahead and freezer friendly dip is a total breeze to put together. All you need is a bag of dried beans to indulge in this smooth, tasty and delicious dip. The lusciously fragrant soft black beans make for a great healthy dish.

Servings: 24

Ingredients

1½ cups black beans, dried
1 can crushed or diced tomatoes
1 ¾ cup vegetable broth
2 medium jalapenos, chopped and diced
1 medium onion, diced
4 cloves garlic, minced
1 lime, juice
1½ tablespoons avocado oil
1 teaspoon smoked paprika
2 teaspoons ground cumin
½ teaspoon ground coriander
½ teaspoon chili powder
¾ teaspoon sea salt

Topping Options

Cilantro
Salsa
Greek Yogurt
Sour cream
Guacamole
Pico de Gallo
Diced bell pepper
Sliced jalapenos
Chopped red onion
Chopped tomatoes

Instructions

1. Rinse the black beans and place them in the Instant Pot.
2. Add the chopped veggies, minced garlic, lime juice, oil, spices and broth into the pot and stir them.
3. Press the "Bean" button and set the timer to cook for 30 minutes at "High Pressure."
4. Once the timer goes off, allow Natural Pressure Release for 10 minutes then do a Quick Pressure Release for the remaining pressure.
5. Place the dish in a blender or food processor and blend it into a smooth and creamy mixture. Add a spicy kick to your dip by adding red pepper flakes, hot sauce, spicy salsa or cayenne.
6. Serve with your favorite toppings and enjoy!

Sweet and Spicy Meatballs

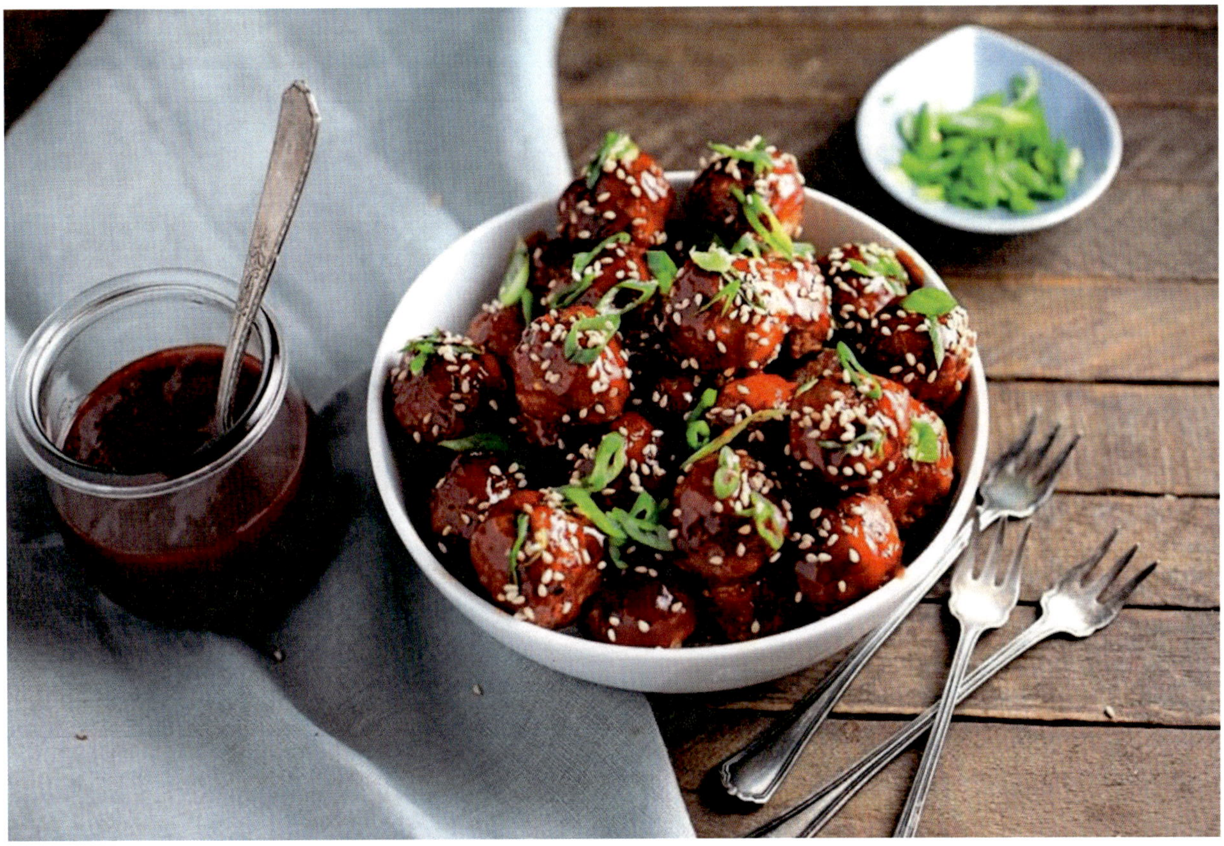

Prep Time: 15 minutes. Cook Time: 10 minutes. Total Time: 25 minutes.

These Instant Pot meatballs are the perfect blend of sweet, smoky and spicy and are sure to become a favorite appetizer. Sweet and Spicy Meatballs is a delicious, easy and quick to make dish.

Servings: 8-10

Ingredients

16 ounces Cooked perfect meatballs (or the brand or flavor available at your local grocery store)
½ cup water
12oz grape jelly
12oz chili sauce
½ tablespoon crushed red pepper
½ teaspoon cayenne pepper

Optional

1 green onion, chopped for garnish

Instructions

1. Place the meatballs in the Instant Pot.
2. Combine grape jelly, chili sauce, spices and water in a medium mixing bowl and stir the mixture.
3. Pour the mixture over the meatballs and combine the mixture.
4. Seal the lid. Set the Instant Pot to "Manual" function and set the cook time to 10 minutes.
5. Once the timer goes off, you can either do a Quick Pressure Release or Natural Pressure Release. Let the meatballs sit on "Keep Warm" function.
6. Garnish with the chopped green onions and serve.
7. Enjoy!

Honey Garlic Chicken Wings

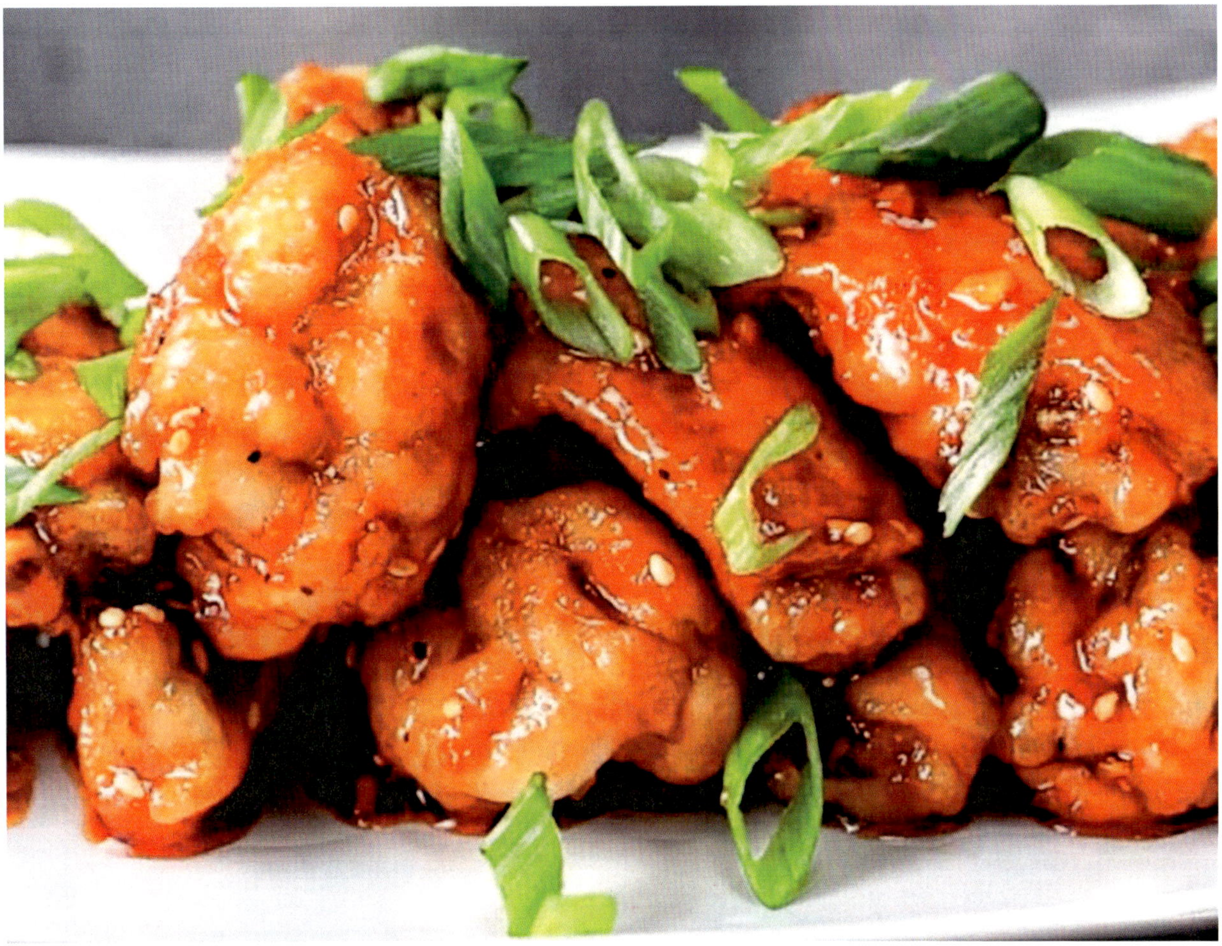

Prep Time: 10 minutes. Cook Time: 20 minutes. Total Time: 30 minutes.

Chicken wings are the ultimate appetizer dish. It's one of those simple yet so delicious finger foods that people can't just get enough. Instant Pot Honey Garlic Chicken Wings are tender and full of flavor. You will enjoy the fragrant and sweet honey marinade. Honey Garlic Chicken Wings are a perfect easy-and-quick-to-make, healthy and kid-friendly dish.

Servings: 2-4

Ingredients

- 1½ pound chicken wings
- ½ cup warm water
- 1-2 Star anise
- 1 small shallot or ½ large shallot, minced
- 4 cloves garlic, minced
- 1½ tablespoon cornstarch
- 1 tablespoon peanut oil

1 tablespoon honey
1 tablespoon ginger, sliced

Chicken wings marinade

1 tablespoon dark soy sauce
2 tablespoons light soy sauce
1 tablespoon Shaoxing wine
¼ teaspoon salt
1 teaspoon sugar

Instructions

1. Mix the marinade ingredients and marinate the chicken wings for about 20 minutes.
2. Add 1 tablespoon of peanut oil in the Instant Pot
3. Set the Instant Pot to "Sauté" function and wait until the indicator displays "Hot" before placing the marinated chicken wings in the pot. This prevents the chicken wings from sticking to the bottom of the pot.
4. Brown/sear the chicken on each side for about a half a minute. Flip a few times before setting them aside. Don't discard the chicken marinade yet.
5. Press the "Cancel" button on the Instant Pot control panel and set it to "Sauté" function. Reduce the heat to "Medium" and add the shallot, ginger and star anise. Stir this combination for about a minute before adding garlic.
6. With a wooden spoon use a mixture of ½ cup of warm water and 1 tablespoon of honey to deglaze the bottom of the pot.
7. Place the chicken wings and leftover marinade back in the Instant Pot. Seal and cook at "High Pressure" for 5 minutes.
8. Allow Natural Pressure Release once the timer goes off and then carefully open the lid. Taste the chicken wings to season with more honey or salt.
9. Remove the chicken wings from the Instant Pot and set them aside. To thicken the Honey Soy Sauce, turn the heat to "Medium" and set the Instant Pot to the "Sauté" function. Add 1 tablespoon of cold water and 1½ tablespoon of cornstarch in the pot and mix into the honey soy sauce. Keep mixing until you reach the desired thickness.
10. Turn off the Instant Pot then return the chicken wings back into the Instant Pot. Thoroughly cover the chicken wings with the honey sauce.
11. Immediately serve and enjoy!

Brisket Sliders Topped with Caramelized Onions

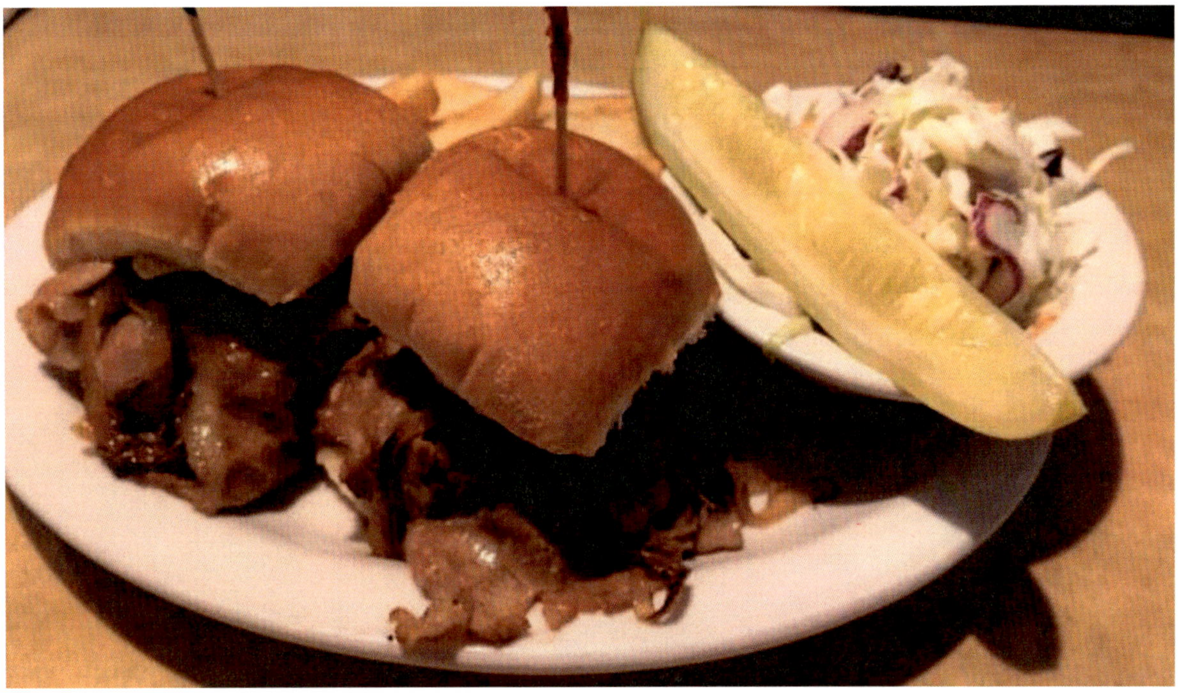

Prep Time: 10 minutes. Cook Time: 50 minutes. Total Time: 1 hour.

Sliders stuffed with tender cooked brisket topped with cheese and caramelized onions are a perfect finger food for backyard parties during the summer. Kids always love the size of these sliders.

Servings: 6

Ingredients

12 slider buns
1½ lbs brisket
6 slices provolone cheese
2 cups beef broth
¼ cup butter, melted
2 onions, caramelized
2 tablespoons olive oil
¼ cup barbeque sauce
1 tablespoon liquid smoke
1-2 tablespoons beef spice rub
½ teaspoon garlic powder
½ teaspoon onion powder

Instructions

1. Season the brisket with beef spice rub and refrigerate for about 30 minutes.

2. Program the Instant Pot to "Sauté" setting and add olive oil. Take out the brisket from the refrigerator and sear it. Turn the fatty side of the brisket up then pour in the beef broth and add in the liquid smoke. Seal the lid.
3. Program the Instant Pot to "Manual" function and cook on "High Pressure" for 50 minutes. Allow Natural Release when the cook time lapses.
4. Carefully remove the brisket and set it on a plate. Shred the brisket and set aside.
5. Preheat the oven. Place the buns on a baking dish and top with the shredded brisket, caramelized onions, barbeque sauce, cheese and finally cover with a top bun.
6. Mix the garlic powder, onion powder and melted butter in a small mixing bowl then rub the mixture over the buns.
7. Bake for about 10-minutes until the cheese completely melts, and the buns are golden brown.
8. Serve and enjoy.

Buffalo Chicken Lettuce Wraps

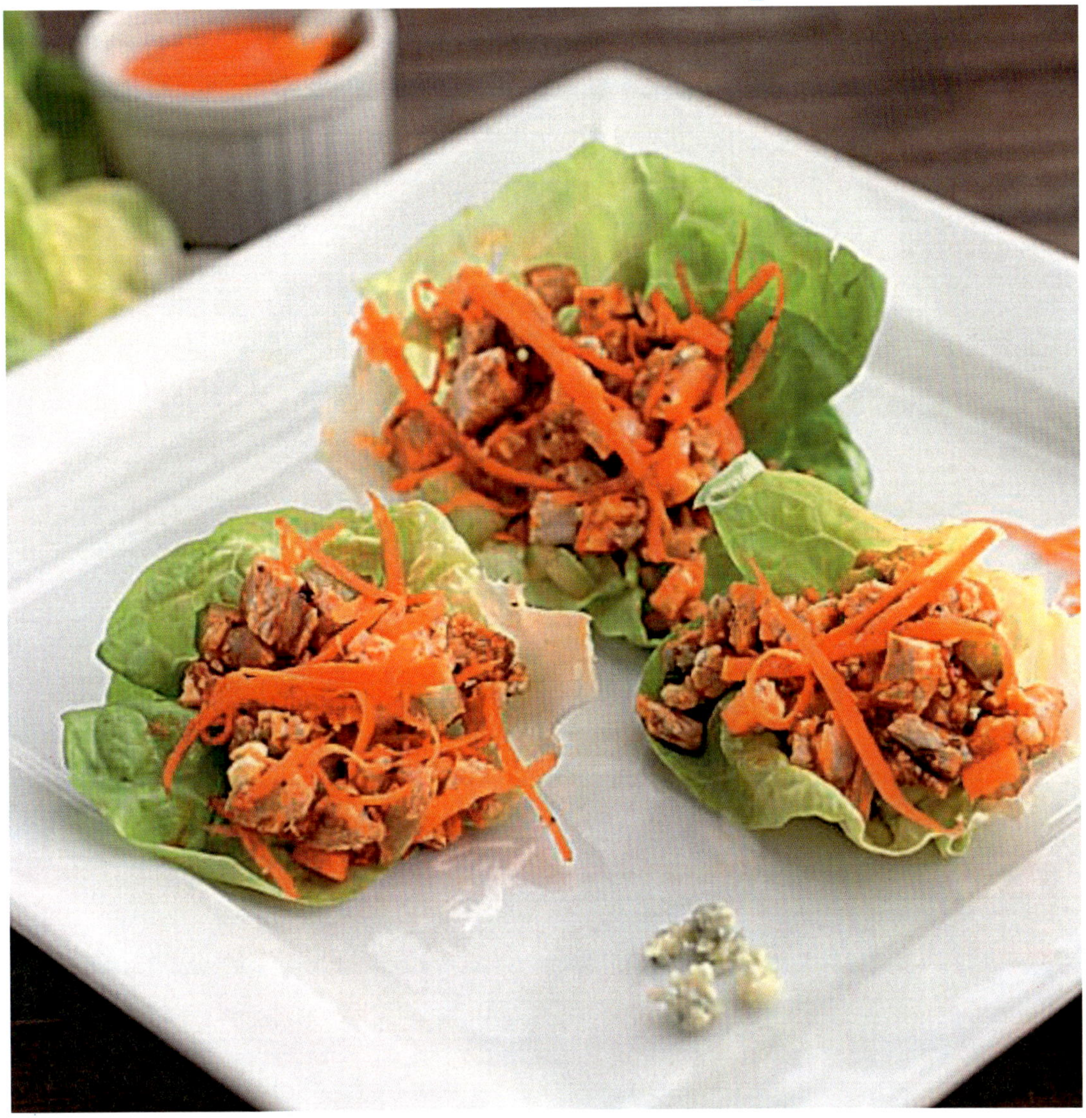

Prep Time: 10 minutes. Cook Time: 18 minutes. Total Time: 28 minutes.

This Buffalo Chicken Lettuce Wraps perfectly combines all the delicious flavors from buffalo wings minus the added fat. Other than wraps, use the shredded chicken in sandwiches, salads and pizza toppings.

Servings: 6

Ingredients

Chicken

24 oz chicken breast, skinless and boneless
16 oz low sodium chicken broth
½ cup hot cayenne pepper sauce
½ onion, finely diced
1 clove garlic
1 celery stick

Wraps

6 lettuce leaves, Iceberg or Bibb
2 large celery stalks, cut into 2-inch pieces
1½ cups carrots, shredded

Instructions

1. Place the chicken, onions, celery stalk and garlic in the Instant Pot. Pour in enough chicken broth to cover the chicken.
2. Seal the lid. Program the Instant Pot to cook at "High Pressure" for 15 minutes.
3. Allow Natural Release once the timer goes off. Carefully open the lid and set aside the chicken. Reserve ½ a cup of the broth, then discard the rest.
4. Shred the chicken into pieces and place it back into the Instant Pot and pour in the reserved ½ cup broth and the hot cayenne pepper sauce.
5. Program the Instant Pot to "Sauté" function and cook for about 2-3 minutes.
6. In each lettuce leaf place ½ cup buffalo chicken and ¼ cup celery and shredded carrots. Use any of your desired dressing, wrap up and serve.
7. Enjoy!

Teriyaki Wings

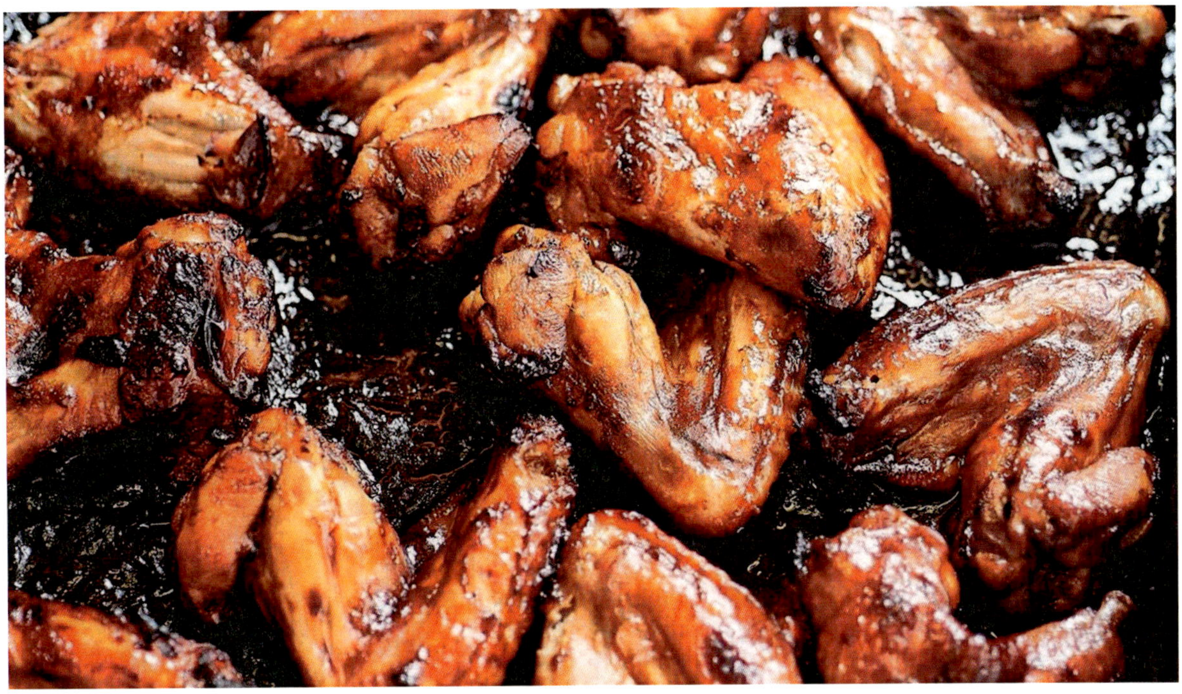

Prep Time: 5 minutes. Cook Time: 35 minutes. Total Time: 40 minutes

Instant Pot Teriyaki Wings are a finger-licking appetizer and an excellent make-ahead dish. The Asian flavors are sure to excite your taste buds and excite your dinner guests.

Servings: 20 wings

Ingredients

2 ½ lb chicken wings
1/3 cup sugar
½ cup soy sauce
2 tablespoons green onions, sliced
1-2 teaspoons sesame seeds, toasted
1 tablespoon water
1 tablespoon cornstarch
1 tablespoon vegetable oil
1 teaspoon sesame oil
2 tablespoons rice wine vinegar
2 tablespoons ginger, grated or minced
2 tablespoons garlic, minced
¼ teaspoon cinnamon powder
1 teaspoon sriracha sauce
½ teaspoon freshly ground black pepper

Instructions

1. Add sesame oil, sugar, freshly ground pepper, ginger, cinnamon, rice vinegar, soy sauce and sriracha sauce in an inner pot. Stir together the ingredients then add the chicken wings. Stir to coat the chicken wings and close the lid.
2. Program the Instant Pot to cook at "High Pressure" for 5 minutes.
3. Line a baking pan with foil and grease it with vegetable oil while the chicken wings cook.
4. Once the Instant Pot timer goes off, allow Natural Pressure Release for about 15 minutes then do a Quick Release.
5. Carefully open the lid and place the teriyaki chicken wings on the prepared baking pan.
6. Set the Instant Pot to "Sauté" function and let the teriyaki sauce simmer.
7. In a small mixing bowl combine water and cornstarch into a smooth paste. Stir in the smooth paste into the teriyaki sauce. Stir the sauce for 2-3 minutes to thicken it to your desired consistency. Turn of the Instant Pot.
8. Baste the wings with teriyaki sauce and place the baking pan under a broiler for 15 minutes. Turn the chicken wings to baste the other side with teriyaki sauce when they are halfway through.
9. Garnish with sliced green onions and toasted sesame seeds. You can also serve your Teriyaki Wings with the sauce.
10. Enjoy!

Red Beans and Rice

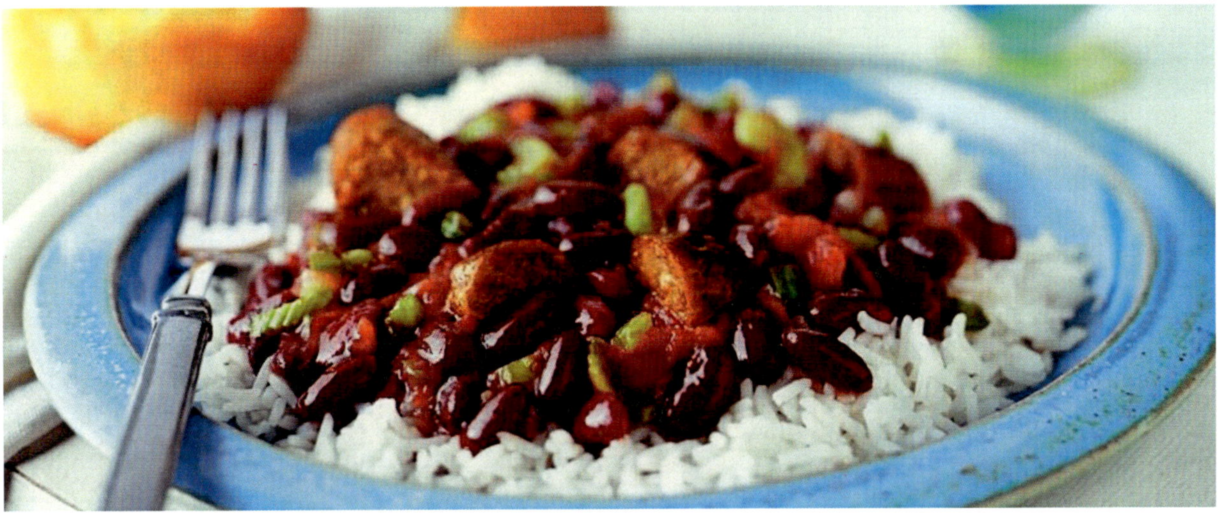

Prep Time: 10 minutes. Cook Time: 43 minutes. Total Time: 53 minutes.

This recipe is normally known for cooking slow and long. However, with an Instant Pot, you will have the Red Bean and Rice recipe ready and served in a little over an hour. You don't have to wait the whole day anymore to enjoy this flavorful dish, and the best part is that you don't even need to presoak the beans. The Instant Pot beans are freezer-friendly, and all you need is a fresh batch of rice to serve this delicacy over and over.

Servings: 10

Ingredients

1 lb red kidney beans, dry
10 cups rice, cooked
1 lb chicken andouille sausage, thinly sliced
7 cups water
1 medium onion, diced
3 cloves garlic, finely minced
3 celery stalks, diced
1 bell pepper, diced
2 bay leaves
1 teaspoon hot sauce
½ teaspoon dried thyme (1 teaspoon fresh thyme)
½ teaspoon black pepper
1 teaspoon salt

Optional

¼ teaspoon white pepper

Instructions

1. Add all the other ingredients in the Instant Pot except the cooked rice and sausage.
2. Seal the lid. Set the Instant Pot to "Manual" function and cook at "High Pressure" for 28 minutes.
3. Once the timer goes off, do a Quick Pressure Release and carefully open the lid.
4. Add the chicken andouille sausage in the pot and re-seal the lid.
5. Program the Instant Pot to "Manual" setting and cook at "High Pressure" for an additional 15 more minutes. When the timer goes off, allow Natural Pressure Release.
6. Let the red kidney beans mixture sit for a while longer in the pot before opening the lid to allow the liquid to thicken.
7. Serve the red kidney beans over a cup of cooked rice.
8. Enjoy!

MAIN COURSE

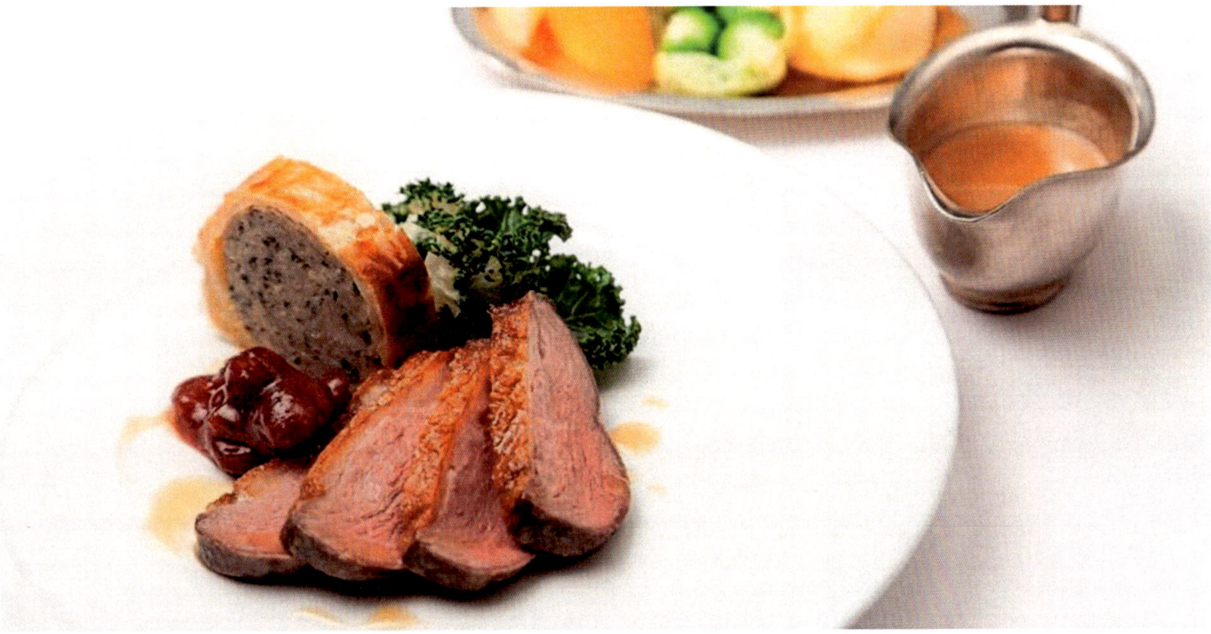

Celebrate the holidays, simply get your family together or host memorable dinner with an Instant Pot comforting home-cooked dinner. Getting dinner on the table is now an easy task with these instant Pot delicious and healthy main dishes which include beef, pork, chicken, fish, pasta and vegetable dishes. These recipes are designed to inspire you whether you are making a simple dinner for the family or entertaining guests. Instant Pot offers quick and easy-to-make dinner recipes as well as healthy inspiration for different cuisines. The key to making an impressive main course dish is choosing the right recipe, to help you here are some of the best Instant Pot main dish ideas. They don't require too much advance prep and they don't take long to cook all you need is to wait for the beeper to go off.

Beef Stroganoff

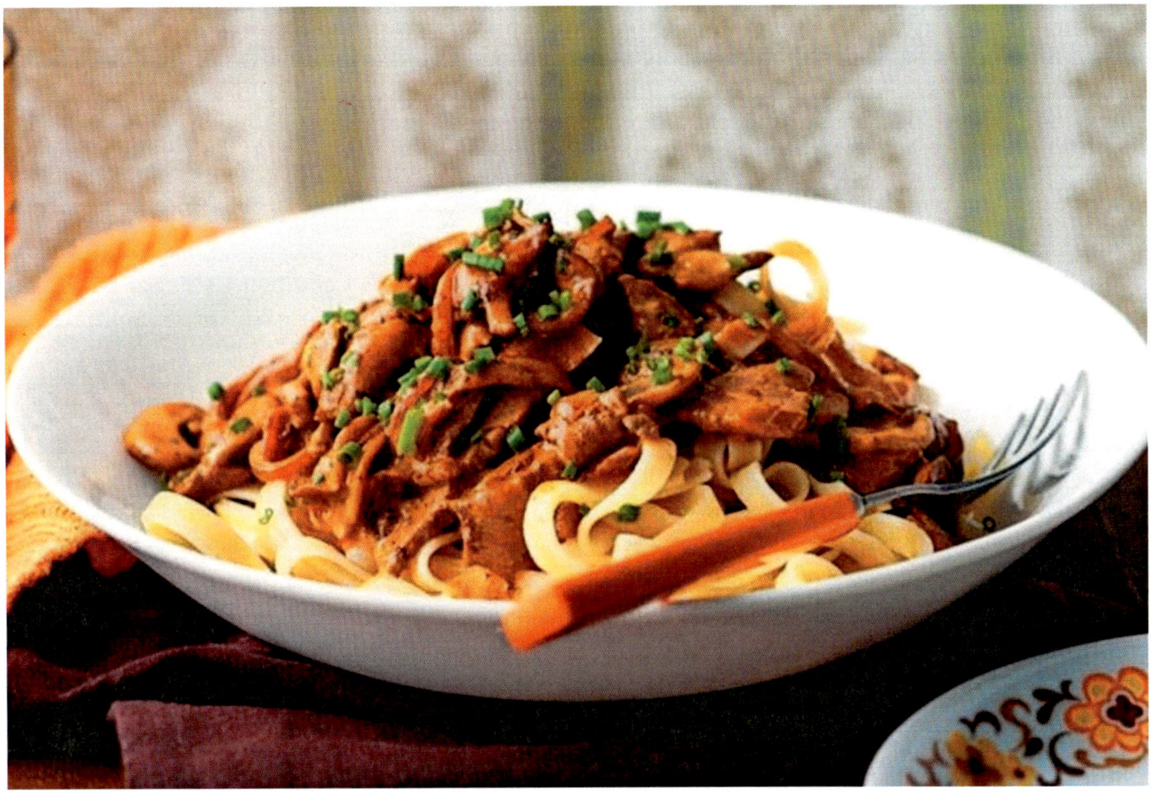

Prep Time: 10 minutes. Cook Time: 44 minutes. Total Time: 54 minutes.

Brace yourself because Instant Pot Beef Stroganoff is about to become a staple dish in your household. It's one of quickest beef stews to make in your Instant Pot. If it's your first time making the dish, the hearty stew of onions, mushrooms, thinly sliced beef steak and sour cream is a real comfort food that everyone enjoys. Beef stroganoff is freezer-friendly making it great for meal prep and batch cooking.

Servings: 3-4

Ingredients

1 lb beef rump steak, thinly sliced into strips
½ lb Swiss, brown or regular white mushrooms
3 cloves garlic, diced
1 large brown onion thinly diced and sliced.
1 cup beef stock
½ cup garden fresh peas (defrost first if frozen)
1/3 cup crème Fraiche or sour cream
1 tablespoon butter or coconut oil
1 tablespoon tomato paste
1 tablespoon yellow mustard or Dijon mustard
½ teaspoon sea salt
1 tablespoon tapioca flour or arrowroot flour or corn flour or rice flour
2 tablespoons flat-leaf parsley, chopped

Pinch of black pepper

Optional

1 bay leaf
Handful porcini mushrooms, dried

Instructions

1. Press the "Sauté" button on the Instant Pot it should cook the dish for 30 minutes on "Normal" heat.
2. Add the coconut oil in the pot, once hot add salt and onion, stir and let it cook for about 2 minutes.
3. Place in the beef strips and continue stirring for another 2 minutes until the meat browns. Add the mushrooms, beef stock, tomato paste, mustard, garlic and bay leaf to the cooking beef strips and stir to combine the ingredients.
4. Press the "Cancel or Keep Warm" button to stop the "Sauté" function then seal the lid. Ensure the steam release valve is set to "Sealing" then program the Instant Pot to "High Pressure" and adjust the timer to 10 minutes.
5. Allow Natural Release for 2-3 minutes after the timer goes off the do a Quick Pressure Release before carefully opening the lid.
6. Press the "Sauté" button. Use a small cup to scoop some stew for dissolving the tapioca flour or any other starch of your choice. Add back the stew to the pot and gently stir through, the stew will thicken. Add the crème Fraiche/sour cream and peas and continue stirring for another minute.
7. Add the parsley and serve with rice pasta, rice or mashed potatoes over steamed veggies.
8. Enjoy.

Faux-tisserie Chicken

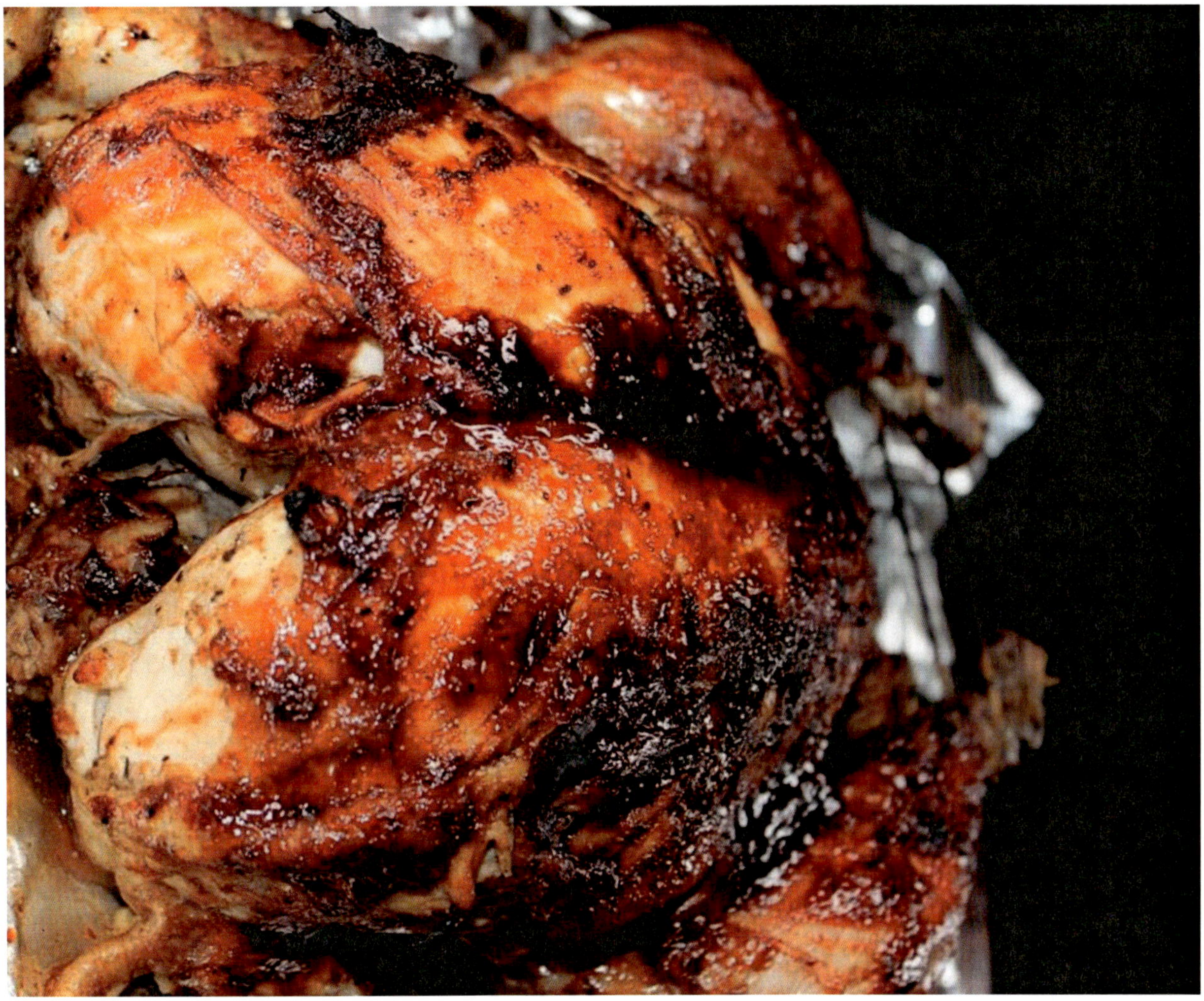

Prep Time: 5 minutes. Cook Time: 33 minutes. Total Time: 38 minutes.

Instant Pot Faux-tisserie Chicken is the healthy and better-tasting alternative to its store-bought equivalent. You are in full control over the seasonings to make pure goodness. Forget the weird sounding ingredients or stuffed brown sugar. For this recipe, you only need garlic, fresh onion, olive oil, and seasonings. Always use a steam rack trivet to avoid the chicken getting soggy. Instead of throwing out garlic and onion, add aromatics, carrots, and celery to make homemade chicken stock.

Servings: 4

Ingredients

2½ - 3lb chicken, whole
5 large cloves fresh garlic, peeled
½ medium onion, diced into quarters
1 cup chicken broth/stock or water
Southwest seasoning mix or 2 tablespoons of your seasoning of choice
2 tablespoons of oil, divided

1 teaspoon onion powder
1 teaspoon chili powder
1 teaspoon garlic powder
½ teaspoon basil
½ teaspoon cumin
Sea salt and black pepper to taste

Instructions

1. Gently rub the chicken with one tablespoon of olive oil and sprinkle with sea salt and freshly black pepper
2. Place the garlic cloves and onion wedges inside the chicken and secure its legs with a butcher's twine.
3. Press "Sauté" button and add a teaspoon of olive oil. Once the oil is hot, place the chicken in the pot. Brown/sear both side for about 4 minutes on every side.
4. Remove the chicken from the pot and set it aside. Place the steam rack in the Instant pot and add the chicken stock to the pot.
5. Sprinkle the seasoning mix over the chicken, rub it in and spread the chicken covering it.
6. Place the chicken on the steam rack with the breast side lying on the rack and seal the lid. Turn the venting valve to "Sealing" position.
7. Program the Instant Pot to "Manual" function and set the timer for 25 minutes.
8. Allow Natural Pressure Release for about 15 minutes once the timer goes off. If need be, do a Quick Release and carefully remove the chicken.
9. Let the chicken rest for about 10 minutes before serving with your favorite side dish.
10. Enjoy!

Indian Butter Chicken

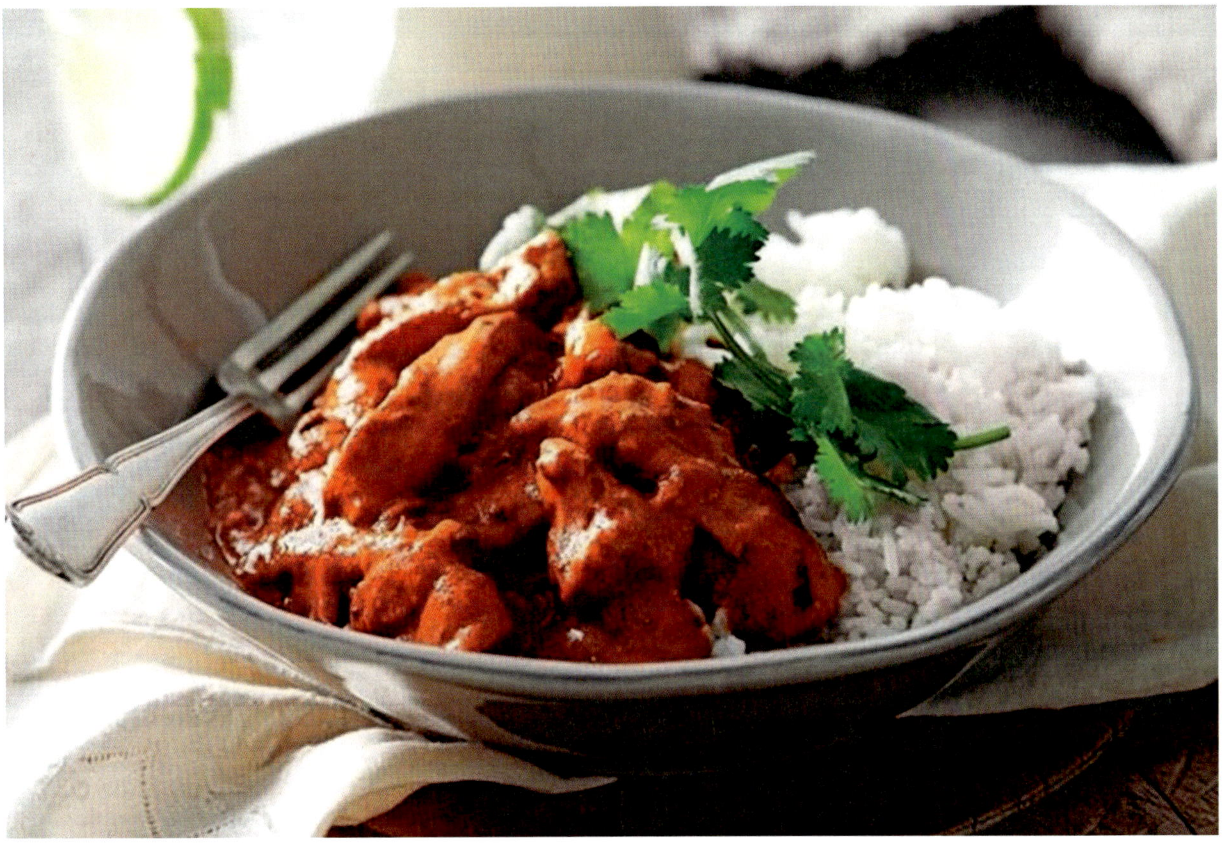

Prep Time: 10 minutes. Cook Time: 15 minutes. Total Time: 25 minutes.

Most home cooks are inspired by different cultures and what cuisine they offer. Experiencing Indian Cuisine through this chicken dish is quite an adventure for the whole family. The Indian Butter Chicken is easy to make in the Instant Pot, and the subtle flavor it carries is sure to get addictive with just a bite.

Servings: 4-6

Ingredients

2 lbs chicken breast or tenderloins (dice into ¼ inch pieces)
1 cup chicken stock
16 oz can tomato paste
1 can coconut milk
½ cup (or 1 stick) butter
1 onion, minced
5 garlic cloves, minced
2 tablespoons cornstarch
1 tablespoon water
2 teaspoons curry powder
2 teaspoons garam masala

2 teaspoons fresh ginger, minced (or 1 teaspoon ground ginger)
1 teaspoon ground cumin
Salt, to taste
Cilantro, for garnishing

Optional

2 teaspoons cayenne pepper

Instructions

1. You can either program the Instant Pot to "Sauté" mode or "Chicken/Meat."
2. Place the stick of butter in the Instant Pot and let it melt until gets foamy with an amazing aroma.
3. Add garlic and onions in the pot, once they are halfway done add the chicken stock, coconut milk, and tomato paste. Stir thoroughly to mix the combination before adding the garam masala, curry powder, ginger, ground cumin, salt and cayenne pepper (if desired).
4. Place the thawed or frozen chicken in the pot and seal the lid. Set Instant Pot to cook on "Manual" mode for 15 minutes or use the "Chicken/Meat" mode to cook the meal.
5. Once the timer goes off, allow Natural Pressure release for 10 minutes. You can do a Quick release to remove all the excess steam before carefully removing the lid.
6. If the chicken wasn't diced set the Instant Pot to "Sauté" or "Keep Warm" mode and use a fork and a sturdy spoon to shred or gently cut the chicken into the desired pieces
7. Add a mixture of water and cornstarch into the pot and stir until the sauce thicken
8. Serve the Indian butter chicken on a bed of jasmine rice or basmati rice and garnish with fresh cut cilantro.
9. Enjoy!

Meatloaf and Mashed Potatoes

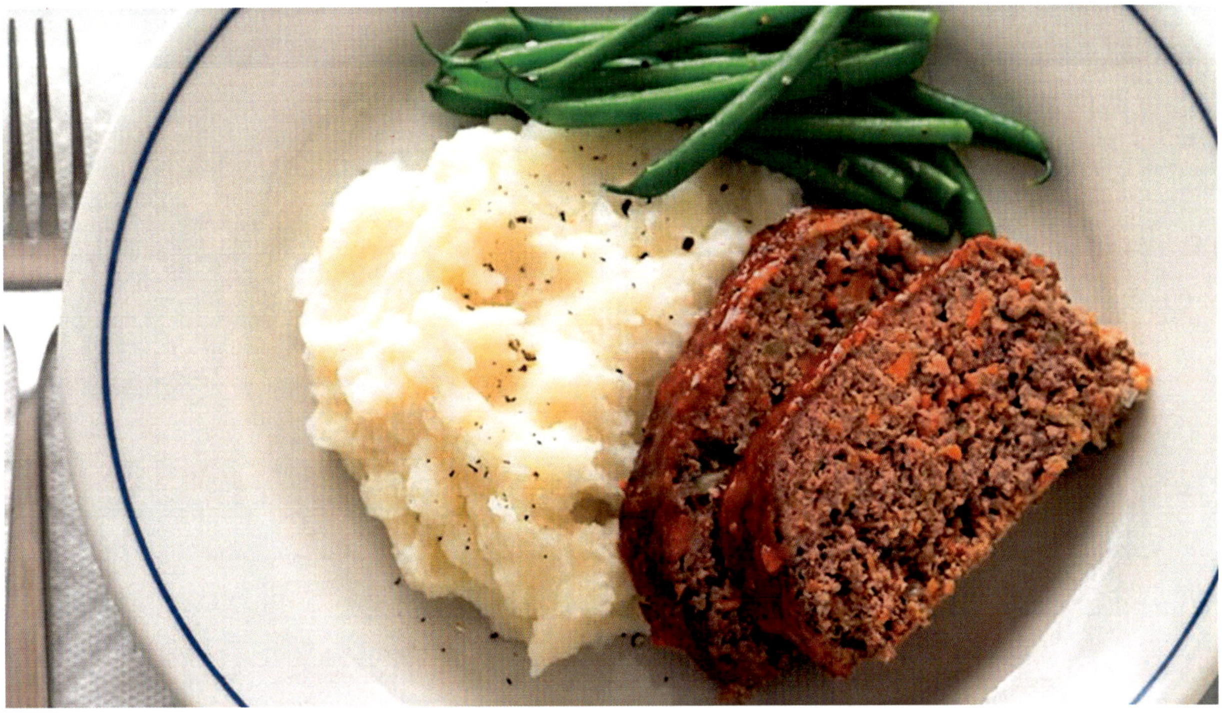

Prep Time: 10 minutes. Cook Time: 25 minutes. Total Time: 35 minutes.

We are always searching for the next delicious, healthy and convenient meal and the Instant Pot Meatloaf and Mashed Potatoes recipe is exactly that. This recipe is cooked in one pot for only 25 minutes. The potatoes come out creamy, and the meatloaf always comes out perfectly moist and tender, never soggy. The best thing about this amazing dish is that you get a quick, delicious filling and you only have a single dish to clean.

Servings: 4-6

Ingredients

Meatloaf

2 pounds ground beef
2 eggs
1 cup dried breadcrumbs
½ cup onion, finely chopped and thinly sliced
2/3 cup ketchup, divided
2-3 fresh garlic cloves, minced
2 teaspoons parsley, dried
2 teaspoons Worcestershire sauce
2 teaspoons salt
½ teaspoon black pepper, freshly ground

Mashed potatoes

3 lbs Yukon gold potatoes, chopped into 1-inch cubes
1 cup chicken broth or water
½ stick (4 tablespoons) unsalted butter
½ cup sour cream
½ cup heavy whipping cream
Freshly ground pepper and kosher salt, to taste

Instructions

1. Place the ground beef, breadcrumbs, eggs, 1/3 cup of the ketchup, Worcestershire sauce, parsley, onion, and garlic in a large bowl and mix the ingredients until they are evenly combined. Place the mixture on disposable loaf pan or fashion one from aluminum foil.
2. In an even layer arrange the potatoes at the bottom of the Instant Pot and then cover them with water or broth. Place the steam rack into the pot and set the meatloaf on top.
3. Seal the lid. Adjust the steam release valve to "Sealed" position and program the Instant Pot to "Manual" function and cook on "High Pressure" for 25 minutes.
4. Do a Quick Pressure Release once the timer goes off and carefully remove the lid.
5. Carefully remove the steam rack with the meatloaf. Drain any excess liquids and brush the meatloaf with remaining ketchup
6. Add sour cream, heavy whipping cream, butter, pepper, and salt to the potatoes and mash them until creamy.
7. Serve and Enjoy!

Taco Pie

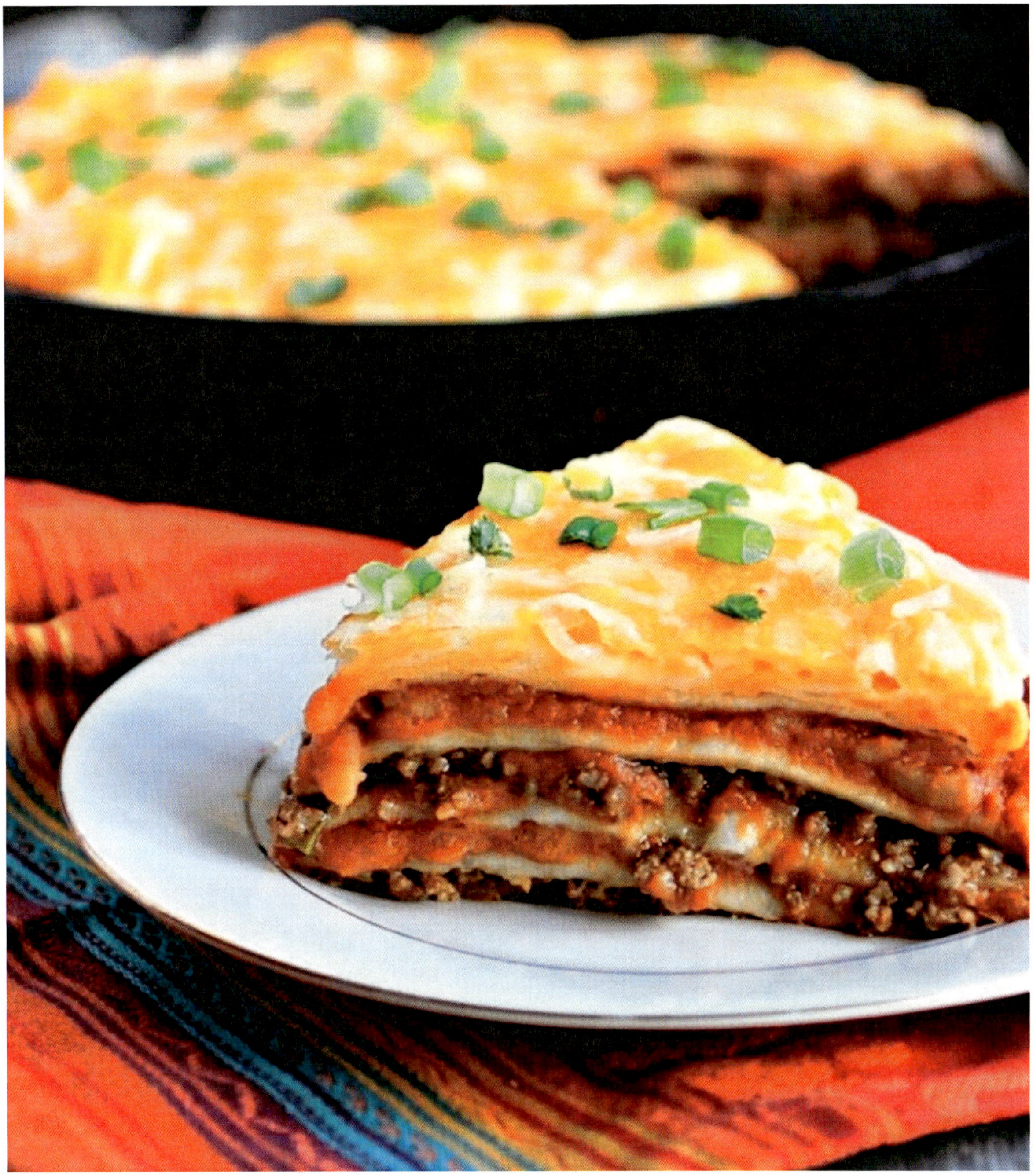

Prep Time: 15 minutes. Cook Time: 25 minutes. Total Time: 40 minutes.

This Taco Pie is a fun layering recipe that is kid-friendly, and family approved. Refried beans, meat, salsa, cheese, and tortillas perfectly come together to make this tasty Mexican pie. You can scale this recipe up or down and tweak it to be cheesier, saucier and even spicier.

Servings: 4-6

Ingredients

- 1 lb lean ground beef or turkey
- 4 flour tortillas (7-8 inches)
- 1½ cups refried beans
- 2 ½ cups shredded cheese
- ½ cup salsa
- 1 oz taco seasoning packet

Optional

- 1/3 cup enchilada sauce

Instructions

1. Program the Instant Pot to "Sauté" mode and add the meat. Brown the meat and stir in the taco seasoning halfway through the browning. When the timer goes off, cancel the "Sauté" setting remove the meat and set it aside.
2. Rinse or wash the pot and add 1½ cups of water into the Instant Pot. Place the trivet in the Instant Pot.
3. Add the refried beans to the salsa and mix.
4. Grease your push pan, springform pan or a cooking pan that fits in your Instant Pot with cooking spray. Place 1 tortilla in the pan and spread over it ½ of the refried bean and salsa mixture. Sprinkle evenly 1 cup of the browned meat then 1/3 cup enchilada sauce if required and 1 cup of cheese.
5. Place the second tortilla in the pan and add the layers of ingredients as on the first tortilla, ½ cup refried bean and salsa mixture, 1 cup of browned meat and ½ cup cheese.
6. Place the third tortilla in the pan and repeat the layering process, ½ cup refried bean and salsa mixture, 1 cup of browned meat and ½ cup of cheese.
7. Place the 4th and final tortilla in the pan and gently press it in place.
8. Cover the pan with foil and place it on top of the steam rack trivet.
9. Close the lid then set the steam release knob to "Sealing" position.
10. Program the Instant Pot to "Manual" function and set a timer for 17 minutes.
11. Allow Natural Pressure Release for about 10 minutes once the timer goes off. Then adjust the steam release knob to "Venting" position to allow the release of the reminder pressure/steam.
12. Carefully open the lid. Use oven mitts to carefully remove both the pan and steam rack/trivet from the Instant Pot. Sprinkle the remaining cheese on the taco pie and brown in the oven (optional).
13. Carefully place the taco pie on a serving plate. Cut it into desired serving sizes and garnish as desired and serve.
14. Enjoy!

Lemon Shrimp Risotto

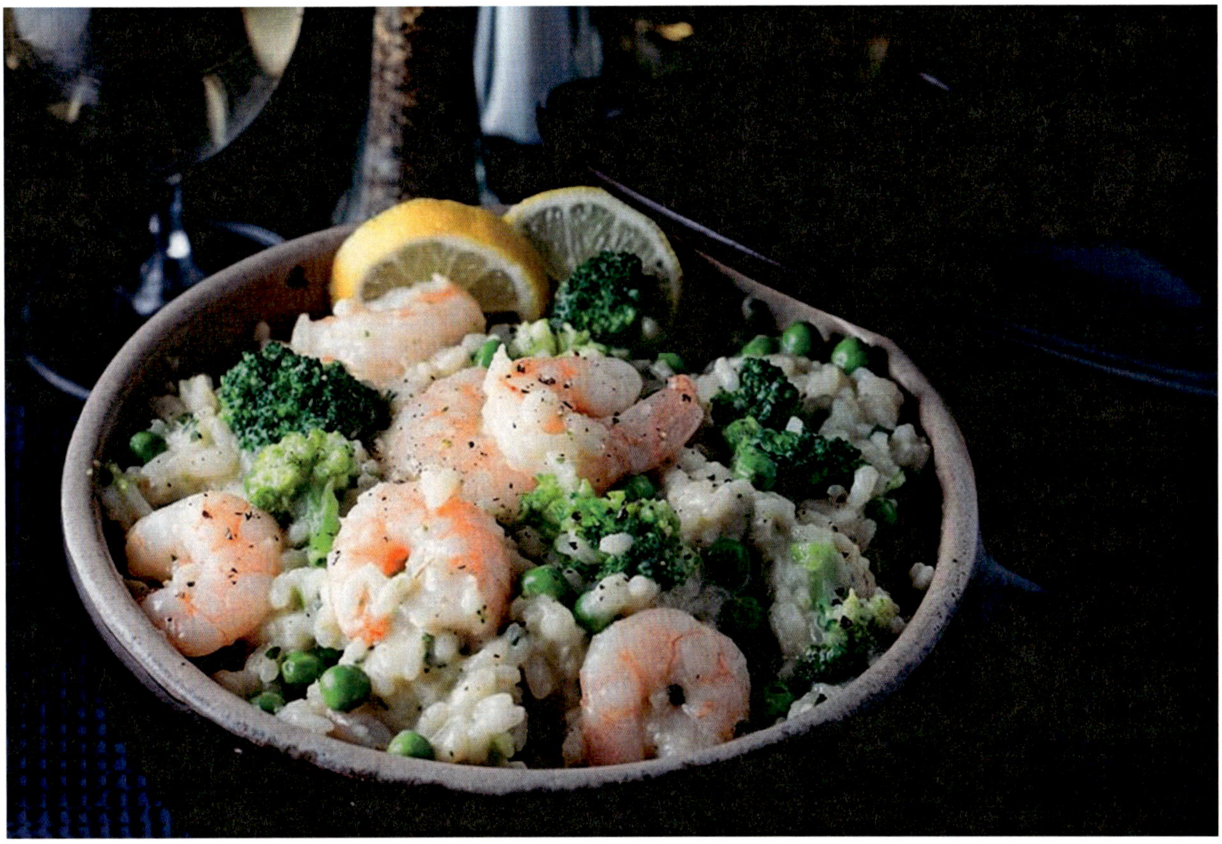

Prep Time: 10 minutes. Cook Time: 15 minutes. Total Time: 25 minutes.

Most rice dishes take almost 30 minutes to cook, but with an Instant Pot, you can make this recipe with a record half that time. This is a great and easy-to-make recipe that perfectly fits an on-the-go-lifestyle. Risotto is a great comfort food and the addition of nutritious green veggies and protein filled shrimp brings out a gourmet feel to this dish.

Servings: 4

Ingredients

1 lb shrimp, peeled and deveined
1½ cups Arborio rice
1 bunch asparagus, thinly sliced
1 cup fresh spinach
3 garlic cloves, minced
½ white onion, chopped
3 ½ cups chicken broth
½ cup Parmesan-Reggiano cheese, shredded
½ cup white wine (Chardonnay or Pinot Grigio)
½ lemon, juice
1 tablespoon butter

2 teaspoons olive oil
1 tablespoon parsley, chopped
Chicken seasoning, salt, and pepper, to taste.

Instructions

1. Program your Instant Pot to the "Sauté" function and wait for about 1 minute for the pot to heat up before adding in the olive oil.
2. Add the chopped asparagus to the pot and cook for about 3 minutes until soft. Remove the asparagus and set aside.
3. Add the onion and garlic in the pot and cook till fragrant.
4. Add butter and wait for it to melt before adding rice to the pot. Stir the rice for about 2 minutes until it's fully coated by the butter.
5. Add the white wine and deglaze the pot with a wooden spoon.
6. Add Parmesan-Reggiano, chicken broth and season the cooking mixture with salt and pepper.
7. Stir thoroughly before sealing the lid. Program the Instant Pot to "Manual" mode and cook at "High Pressure." Set the timer for 8 minutes.
8. As the risotto cooks, prepare and season the shrimp.
9. Do a Quick Pressure Release before carefully removing the lid. Set the Instant Pot to "Sauté" function. Push the risotto to one side of the pot and add the remaining olive oil on the empty side. Place the shrimp and veggies into the empty portion of the pot.
10. Turn the shrimp to cook on both sides for about 3-4 minutes until its pink and spinach are wilted.
11. Stir thoroughly to combine all the items in the pot. Drizzle fresh lemon juice and sprinkle the parsley on the dish.
12. Remove from the Instant Pot and let it cool before serving.
13. Enjoy!

Salmon with Chili Lime Sauce

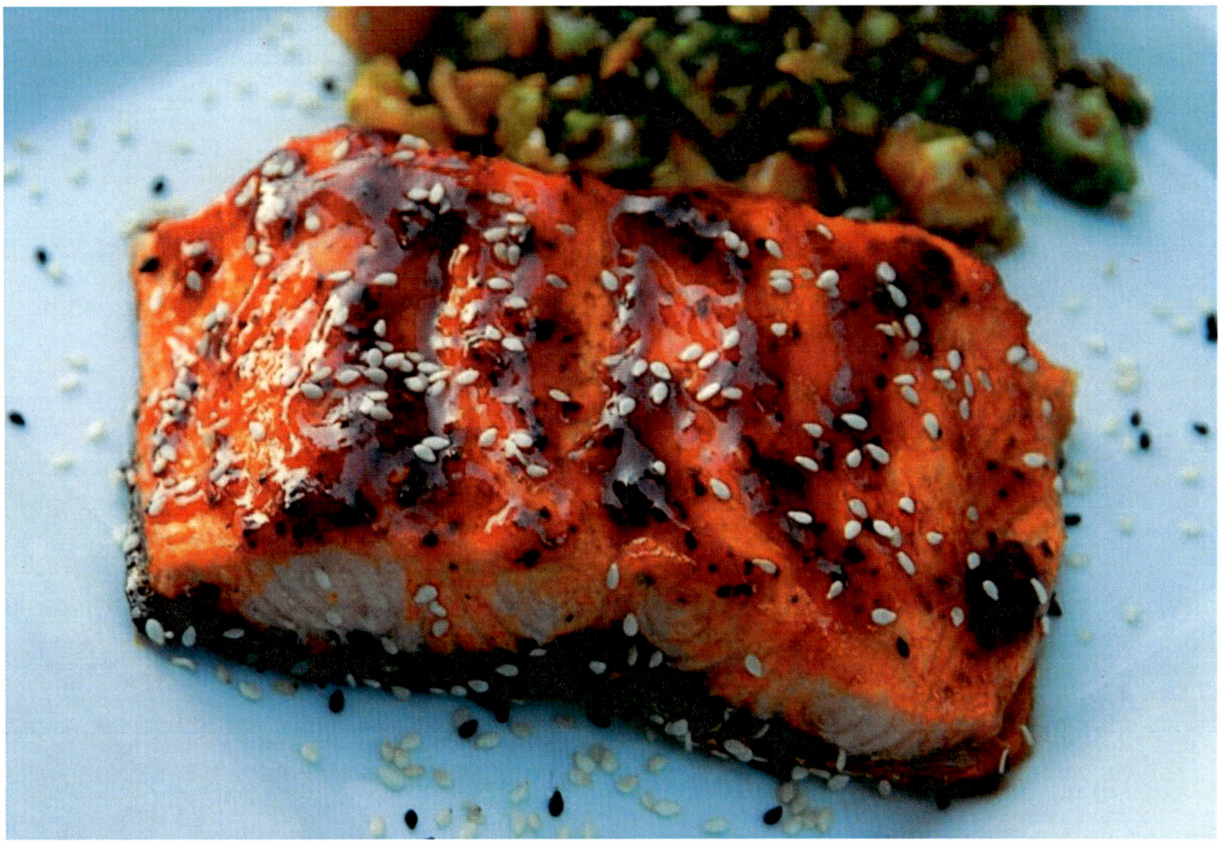

Prep Time: 10 minutes. Cook Time: 5 minutes. Total Time: 15 minutes.

Make any perfect seafood dish in just 5 minutes in the Instant Pot. This Instant Pot Salmon recipe cooks fast just have the accompanying side dish ready before you pop the salmon in the Instant Pot. So, make the chili-lime sauce ready first because it will take longer to cook than the salmon.

Servings: 2

Ingredients

Salmon

2 (5oz each) salmon fillets
1 cup water
Freshly ground black pepper and sea salt, to taste

Chili-lime sauce

1 jalapeno, seeded and diced
2 cloves garlic, minced
1 lime juiced
1 tablespoon olive oil
1 tablespoon hot water

1 tablespoon honey
1 tablespoon fresh parsley, chopped
½ teaspoon cumin
½ teaspoon paprika

Instructions

1. Combine all the chili-lime sauce ingredients and mix them in a bowl and set it aside.
2. Add water to the Instant Pot and place the steam rack in the pot. Place the salmon fillet on the steam rack.
3. Season the salmon fillets with pepper and salt to your liking.
4. Cover and seal the lid. Set the Instant Pot to "Steam" function, "High Pressure" and set the cook time to 5 minutes.
5. Once the timer goes off, do a Quick Pressure Release and carefully open the lid.
6. Place the salmon on a serving plate and generously drizzle with the chili-lime sauce.
7. Serve and Enjoy!

Easy Macaroni and Cheese

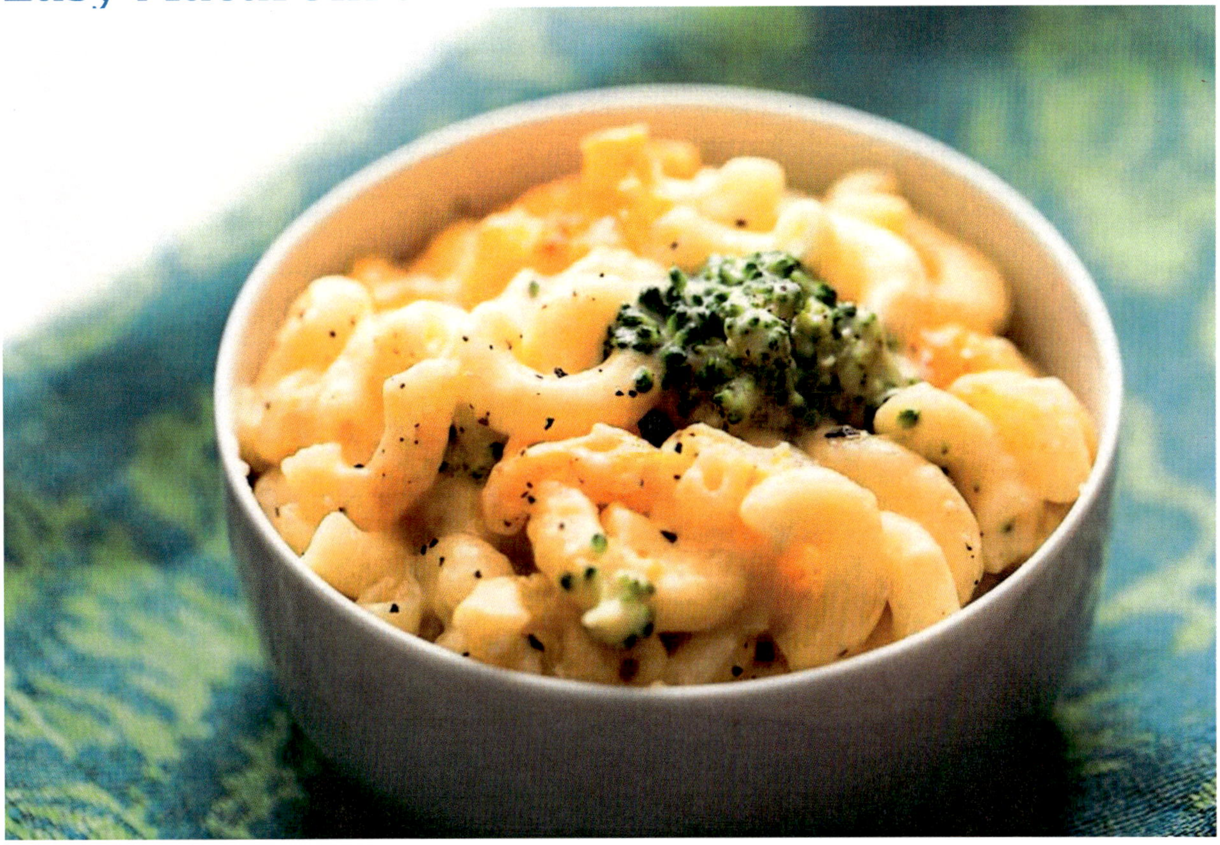

Prep Time: 5 minutes. Cook Time: 5 minutes. Total Time: 10 minutes.

Forget the usual boxed mac and cheese. Make this kid-friendly dish in the Instant Pot in record time. The Instant Pot Mac and Cheese is a cheesy, delicious and creamy, perfect weeknight meal for the whole family. And it tastes way better than the boxed stuff.

Servings: 6-8

Ingredients

1 lb elbow macaroni
½ parmesan cheese
8 oz sharp cheddar cheese
8 oz Monterey jack cheese
1 cup evaporated milk
4 cups water
4 tablespoons butter
2 teaspoon ground mustard
½ teaspoon black pepper
2 teaspoon sea salt or kosher, to taste

Instructions

1. Add macaroni, water, butter, mustard, pepper, and salt in the Instant Pot and seal the lid.
2. Set the Instant Pot to "Manual" setting and cook for 4 minutes on High Pressure. (Cook your macaroni for only 3 minutes on High Pressure if the cook time indicated in the packaging is less than 6 minutes).
3. Do a Quick Pressure Release once the timer goes off and carefully open the lid. If the pasta isn't completely cooked, program the Instant Pot to "Sauté" and let the pot cook for additional 2 minutes until the pasta is cooked through.
4. Finally, add in the evaporated milk and the cheeses to the pot and stir until the pasta mix into a creamy deliciously. Add more salt if desired.
5. Serve hot and enjoy!

Barbacoa Beef

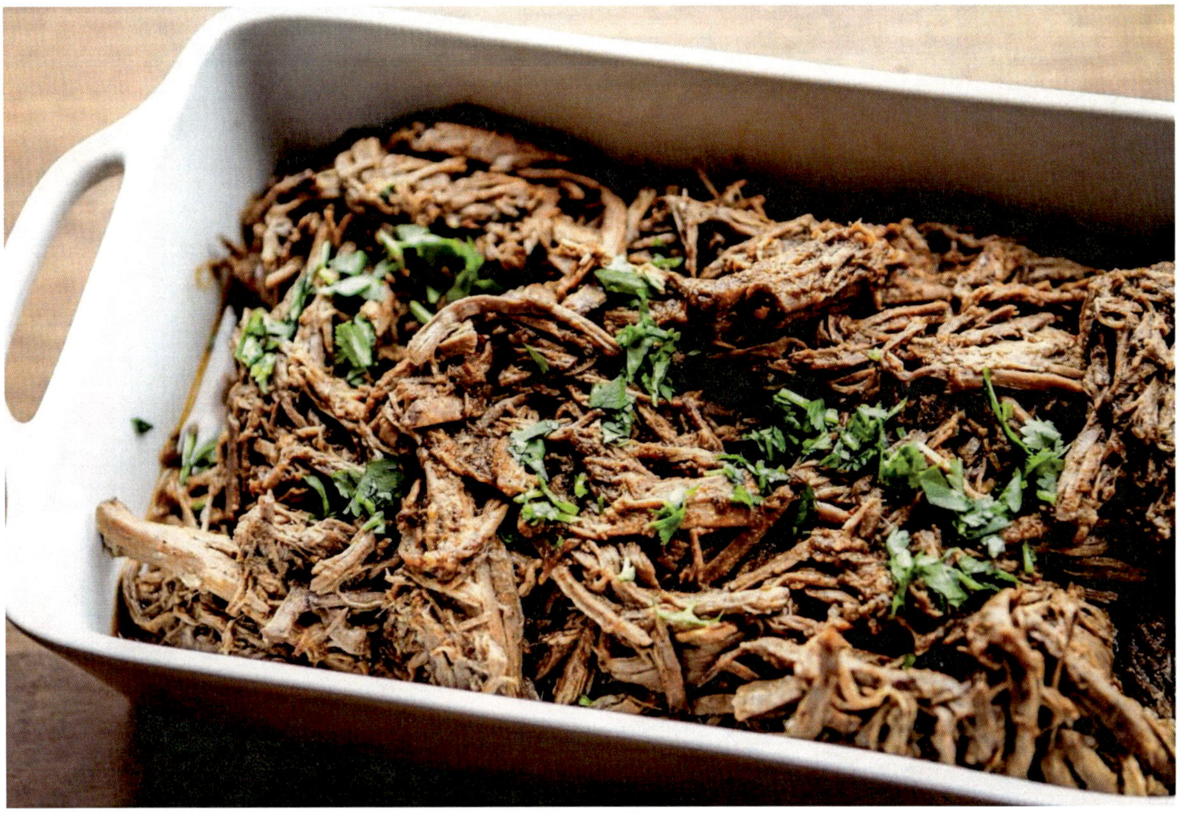

Prep Time: 15 minutes. Cook Time: 1 hour 15 minutes. Total Time: 1 hour 30 minutes.

The Barbacoa Beef recipe may look and use similar ingredients as the Chipotle Shredded Beef recipe, but the two dishes actually taste a lot different than they look served on a plate. This dish is flavorful, bold and spicier and it tastes great served with burritos, enchiladas and tacos. The Instant Pot is a great time saver when it comes to making Barbacoa beef.

Servings: 6

Ingredients

2 lbs chuck roast
½ cup beef broth
¼ cup lime juice, fresh
1 cup yellow onions, finely diced
3 bay leaves
2-4 chipotle chiles, minced, seeded and in adobo sauce
3 cloves garlic, finely minced
1 tablespoon vegetable oil
2 tablespoon apple cider vinegar
1 tablespoon dried oregano
1 tablespoon ground cumin

¼ teaspoon ground cloves
1 teaspoon pepper
2 teaspoons salt

Instructions

1. Remove the large pieces of fat from the chuck roast and cut it into about 4 to 6 chunks.
2. Program the Instant Pot to "Sauté" setting then place half of the cut roast chunks into the pot. Completely sear both sides of the meat and set aside. Repeat the same procedure by searing the remaining half of the meat and setting it aside.
3. Add the onions to the Instant Pot and cook them for about 3 minutes until they are soft and translucent. Add the oregano, garlic, and cumin to the cooked onions and let the combination cook for another minute. Add in the bay leaves, chipotle chiles, cloves, salt, pepper, cider vinegar and pour in the broth and lime juice. Add the seared roast back into the pot and stir to combine.
4. Close the lid. Set the Instant Pot to "High Pressure" and cook for 60 minutes.
5. Once the timer is off, allow Natural Pressure Release and carefully open the lid. Use a pair of tongs to remove the cooked meat and place the chunks on a cutting board and shred the meat into smaller pieces. Return the shredded pieces into the Instant Pot and stir for a few minutes.
6. Serve with your favorite side dish and enjoy.

Chicken Enchiladas

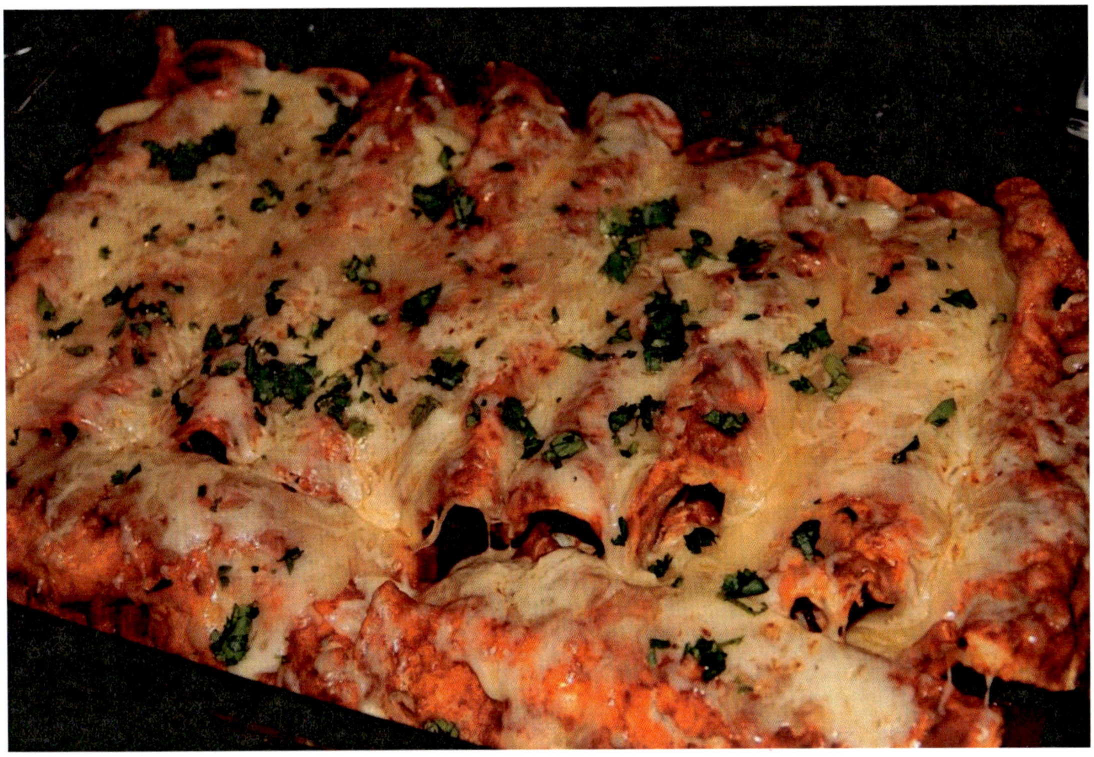

Prep Time: 20 minutes. Cook Time: 20 minutes. Total Time: 40 minutes.

Conveniently make the ever so delicious homemade Chicken Enchiladas in an Instant Pot in just a flash. Easily make the enchilada sauce in the Instant Pot. Compared to the store-bought canned sauce, this homemade enchilada sauce is fresh and full of flavor.

Servings: 12

Ingredients

1½ lbs chicken breasts, skinless and boneless
12 corn tortillas
2 (8oz) cans tomato sauce
8 oz Monterey jack cheese, shredded
8 oz sharp cheddar cheese, shredded
Sour cream
1 cup chicken broth
1 cup onions, finely diced
1 jalapeno, seeded and minced
4 cloves garlic minced
1 tablespoon vegetable oil
2 tablespoons freshly chopped cilantro
2 tablespoons chili powder
1 tablespoon sugar
1 teaspoon cumin
Kosher salt and black pepper, to taste

Instructions

1. Program the Instant Pot to "Sauté" function and heat the vegetable oil. Add the garlic, onions, and jalapeno and sauté for 2-3 minutes, until soft and the onions are translucent
2. Add the sugar, chili powder, cumin, pepper, and salt then pour in the tomato sauce and broth into the Instant Pot and stir to combine the ingredients.
3. Finally, place the chicken in the pot. Close the lid. Ensure the Pressure Release Valve is set to "Sealing" position.
4. Program the Instant Pot to cook on "Manual" setting and cook for 10 minutes.
5. As the sauce and chicken breasts cook, prepare the tortillas.
6. Preheat the oven to 400F. Slightly brush the tortillas with some oil then transfer them to a baking sheet. Place the tortillas in the oven and let them heat for about 5 minutes.
7. Once the timer goes off, do a Quick Release. Carefully open the lid and remove the chicken breast then stir in the chopped cilantro to the sauce. Shred the chicken into sizeable pieces once they cool.
8. Use the non-stick cooking spray to generously grease and coat the baking dish. Pour ¼ a cup of the cooked enchilada sauce into the dish.
9. Divide ½ of the combined the two shredded kinds of cheese, ½ of the remaining enchilada sauce and the shredded chicken pieces among the tortillas. Roll the tortilla up and place them in the baking dish. Ensure the seam side is facing down on the baking dish.
10. Pour all the remaining enchilada sauce into the baking dish. Top the enchiladas with the other ½ of the combined shredded cheeses.
11. Use aluminum foil to cover the baking dish before placing it in an over. At 400F bake the enchiladas for about 20-30 minutes.
12. Once ready sprinkle more freshly chopped cilantro and top with sour cream.
13. Enjoy!

Chicken Pho

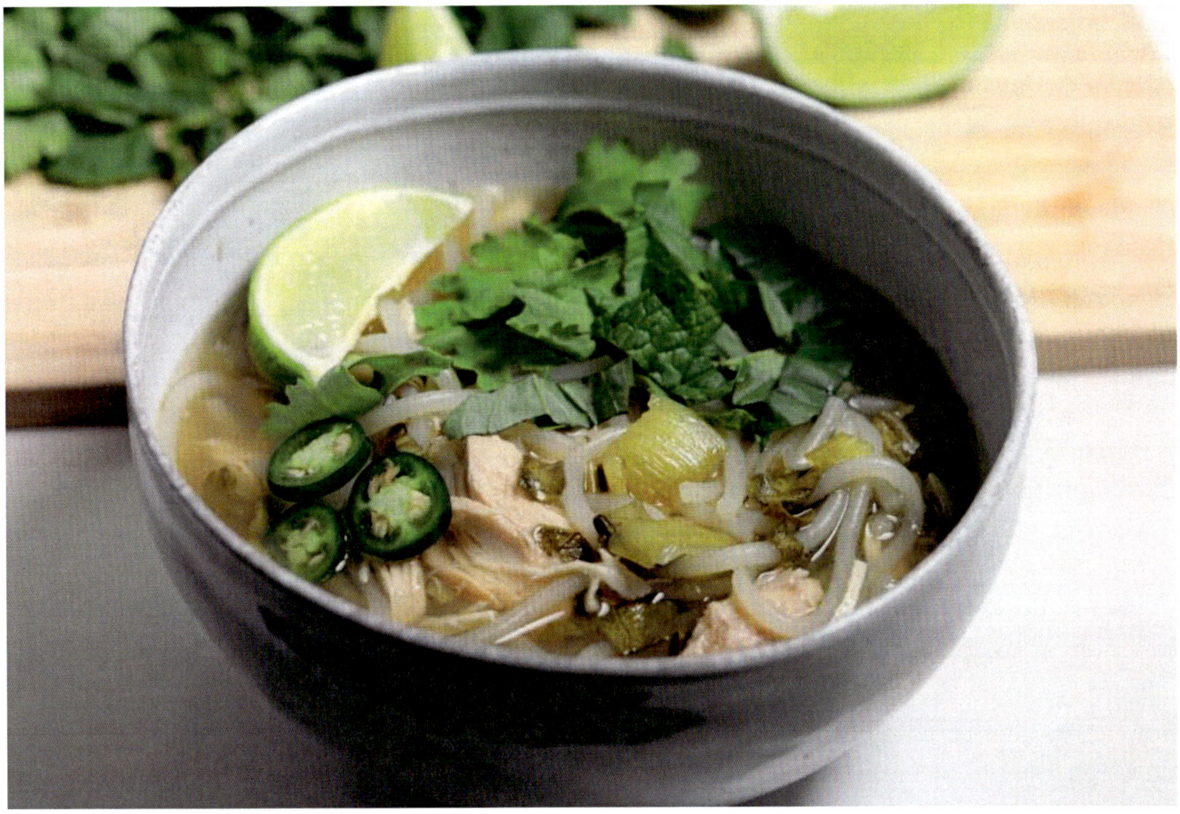

Prep Time: 10 minutes. Cook Time: 30 minutes. Total Time: 40 minutes.

Technically a soup dish, Chicken Pho is a traditional Vietnamese dish can easily be enjoyed as a stand-alone meal. The Instant Pot makes it even easy to make this dish at home.

Servings: 4

Ingredients

6 chicken thighs
14 oz rice noodles
8 cups water
1 large yellow onion, halved
5 cloves
1 cinnamon stick
3 Star anise
3 cardamom pods, smashed
1 Fuji apple, peeled, cored and cut into chunks
1(2-inch) ginger piece, cut into slices and smashed
½ cup chopped cilantro leaves
1 tablespoon olive oil
3 tablespoons fish sauce
1 tablespoon sugar

1 tablespoon coriander seeds
Kosher salt, to taste

Toppings

½ red onion, thinly sliced
Bean sprouts
Fresh herbs of your choice
2 jalapenos, thinly sliced
Sriracha sauce
1 lime, cut to wedges
Daikon radish sprouts

Instructions

1. In a large bowl soak the noodles in warm water for about 30-45 minutes.
2. Program the Instant Pot to the "Sauté" option. Add the oil and wait until it heats before adding ginger and onions. Sauté for about 4 minutes, until charred slightly without stirring.
3. Add the cloves, cinnamon stick, coriander, and star anise into the Instant Pot and cook for an additional minute, until fragrant. Pour in water and add along the chicken, apples, cilantro, sugar and fish sauce.
4. Close the lid and set the Instant Pot to "Manual" setting cook at "High Pressure" for 15 minutes.
5. Allow Nature Pressure Release for approximately 10 minutes once the timer goes off then do a Quick Release to release the remaining pressure.
6. Carefully open the lid, remove the chicken from the pot and set it aside. Strain the broth then season with pepper and salt if desired.
7. Remove the bone from the chicken once it's cool enough to handle. Equally, divide the chicken meat into 4 bowls. Strain the noodles and divide into the bowls then top with the strained broth. Add in any of your desired toppings.
8. Enjoy!

Ham and Penne Pasta

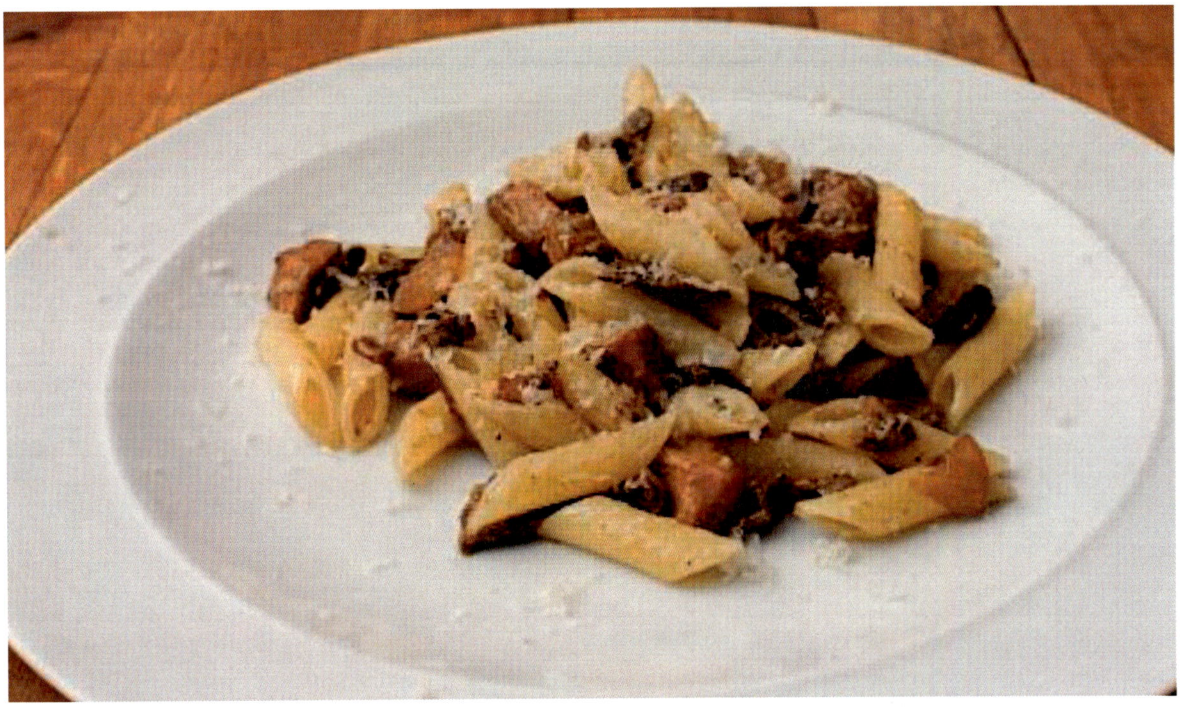

Prep Time: 15 minutes. Cook Time: 8 minutes. Total Time: 23 minutes.

Making Ham and Penne Pasta has gotten way easier with an Instant Pot, and the best part is after this delicious meal you only have one dish to clean up.

Servings: 8

Ingredients

- 3 cups cubed cooked ham
- 1 (16oz) penne noodles, uncooked
- 2 cups frozen peas, thawed
- ¼ cup flour
- ½ cup Parmesan cheese
- 2 cups milk (2%)
- 3 cups chicken broth
- ½ cup yellow onions, diced
- 3 cloves garlic, minced
- 1 tablespoon olive oil
- ½ teaspoon dried basil
- ½ teaspoon dried parsley
- ¼ teaspoon dried oregano
- ¼ red pepper flakes
- ¼ teaspoon pepper

Instructions

1. Turn the Instant Pot to "Manual" function then add olive oil. Sauté the onions and ham for a few minutes, until the onion is soft and translucent. Add the pepper, basil, garlic, oregano, parsley and red pepper flakes into the pot and cook for about 1-2 minutes.
2. Pour in the milk, chicken broth and flour and stir thoroughly until all the ingredients are well combined. Add the rest of the ingredients excluding the parmesan cheese.
3. Close the lid. Program the Instant Pot to cook at "High Pressure" and set the cook time to 8 minutes.
4. Once the timer goes off, allow Natural Pressure Release for about 5 minutes before doing a Quick Release.
5. Sprinkle the Ham and Penne Pasta with Parmesan cheese then serve.
6. Enjoy!

Maple Smoked Brisket

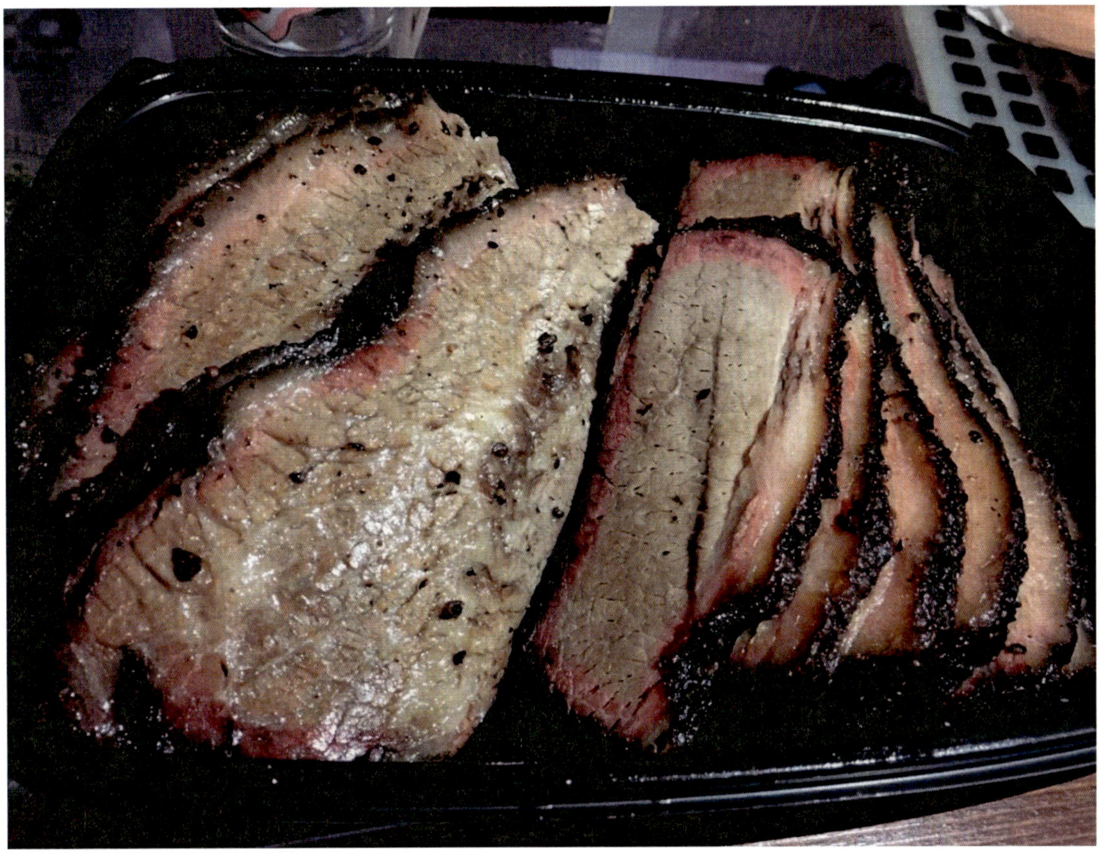

Prep Time: 10 minutes. Cook Time: 1 hour. Total Time: 1 hour 10 minutes.

You don't need an outdoor smoker to enjoy a smoked brisket anymore. All you need is some paprika, smoked sea salt and a little bit of liquid smoke to get that delicious smoky flavor in your Instant Pot.

Servings: 4-6

Ingredients

1½ lbs beef brisket
2 cups bone broth or stock of choice
½ teaspoon smoked paprika
2 teaspoons smoked sea salt
1 tablespoon liquid smoke
3 fresh thyme sprigs
1 teaspoon onion powder
2 tablespoons maple sugar, coconut sugar or date sugar
1 teaspoon mustard powder
1 teaspoon black pepper

Instructions

1. Part dry the brisket with paper towels and set it aside.

2. In a small bowl mix the smoked paprika, smoked sea salt, onion powder, mustard powder, maple sugar, and pepper. Generously coat on both sides of the brisket with the spice blend.
3. Program the Instant Pot to "Sauté" function. Allow the Instant Pot to heat up for about 2-3 minutes. Ensure the bottom of the Instant Pot is greased then place the brisket in the bottom. Sear both sides of the brisket until deeply brown and golden. Turn the brisket so that the fatty side is up before adding thyme, broth, and liquid smoke. Deglaze the pot then close the lid.
4. Press the "Cancel" then reprogram the Instant Pot to "Manual" function and cook at "High Pressure" for 50 minutes.
5. Allow Natural Pressure Release once the timer goes off. Carefully open the lid and remove the brisket. Cover the brisket with foil and allow it to rest.
6. Reset the Instant Pot to "Sauté" function and cook the sauce for 10 minutes, until reduced and thickened.
7. Slice the brisket drizzle with sauce and serve with your favorite side dish and veggies.

Kansas City Style Baby Back Ribs

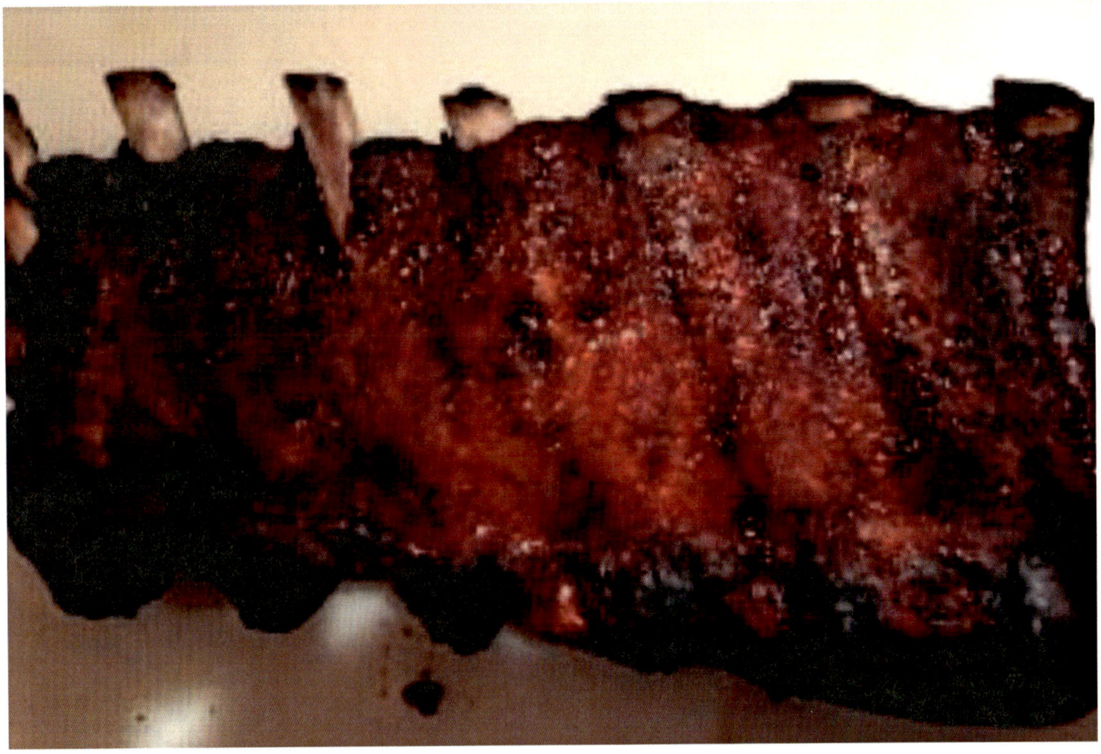

Prep Time: 10 minutes. Cook Time: 28 minutes. Total Time: 38 minutes.

If you love ribs as much as everyone does, then you are going to enjoy the pork baby back ribs in the Instant Pot. It might sound easy, but the dish is amazingly delicious. The Kansas City Style Baby Back Ribs recipe is hands off and takes even lesser time than making them in an oven or over a grill. Enjoy the flavor infused and tender ribs with fresh garden veggies or a full plate of potato salad.

Servings: 4

Ingredients

Ribs and rub
2½ to 3 lbs fresh pork back ribs
1 tablespoon smoked paprika
2 tablespoons dark brown sugar
¾ teaspoon onion powder
¾ teaspoon garlic powder
¼ teaspoon ground red pepper
¾ teaspoon chili powder
¾ teaspoon kosher salt
¾ teaspoon black pepper

Barbecue sauce

¼ cup water
¼ cup ketchup

¼ cup apple cider vinegar
1 tablespoon tapioca

Instruction

1. Part the ribs dry with a paper towel until there is no more moisture is left. Refrigerate the ribs for at least 30 minutes before cooking.
2. Make a spice rub mixture by combining pepper, onion powder, garlic powder, red pepper, paprika, brown sugar, chili powder and salt in a small mixing bowl.
3. Pour a cup of water into the Instant Pot and place a steam rack into the pot. Coil the ribs around so that it fits around the edge of the inner walls of the Instant Pot.
4. Make a homemade barbecue sauce by combining the barbecue ingredients in a small oven safe bowl and place this bowl on the steam rack in the middle of the coiled ribs.
5. Close the lid and ensure the Pressure Releasing Valve is set to "Sealing" position. Program the Instant Pot "Manual" mode and set the cook time for 28 minutes.
6. Once the timer goes off, allow Natural Pressure Release for at least 20 minutes. Carefully open the lid and carefully remove the barbecue sauce and the ribs.
7. Place the ribs on a baking sheet then baste them with the sauce. Place the ribs under the broiler for about 5 minutes then remove and serve.
8. Enjoy!

Spanish Chorizo and Potato Hash

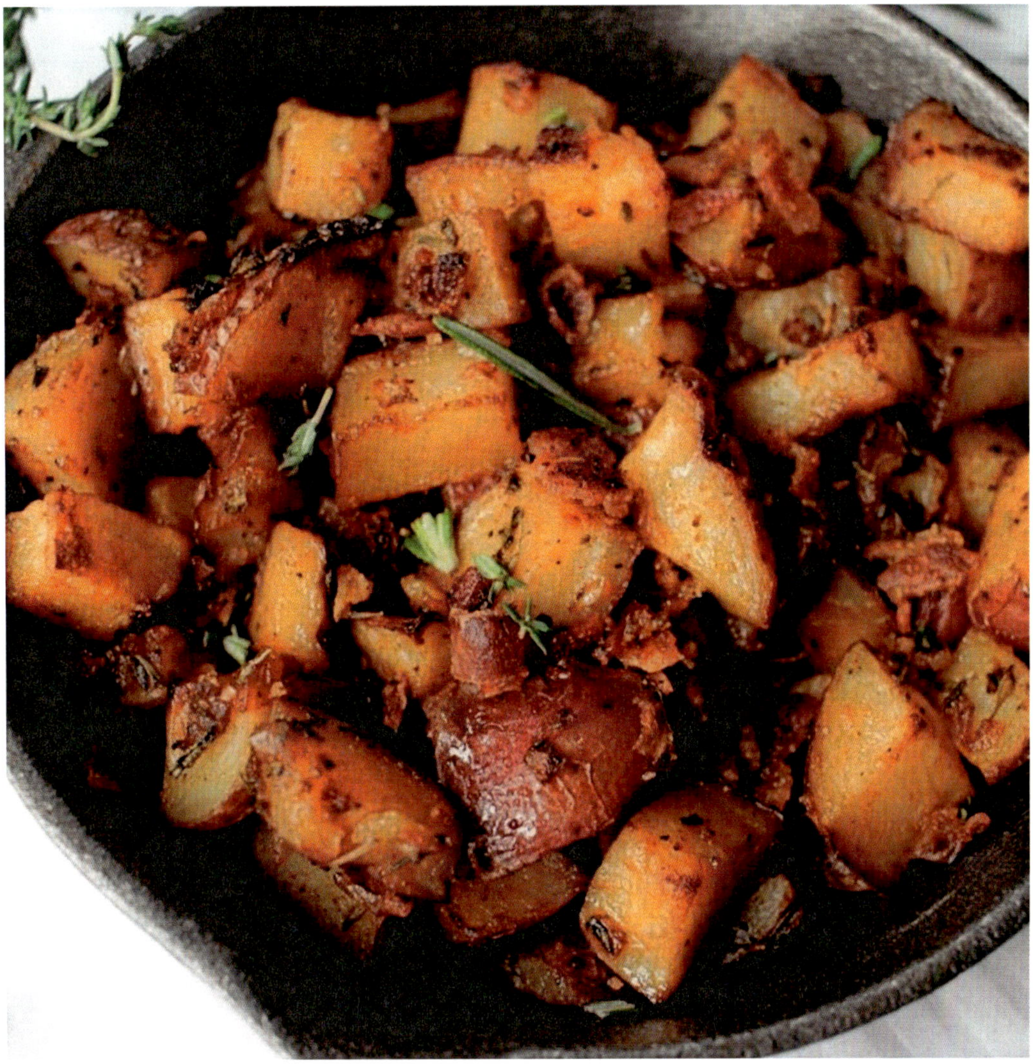

Prep Time: 5 minutes. Cook Time: 15 minutes. Total Time: 20 minutes.

Spanish Chorizo and Potato hash is a delicious opportunity to make use of the leftover dinner potatoes and sausages. Turn the leftovers into a huge potato breakfast dish. This recipe is also a perfect way of impressing your family with the Spanish favorite street food. You can enhance the flavor of your dish by adding rosemary and basil as well as grating some cheddar cheese over the potatoes.

Servings: 4

Ingredients

- 6 large potatoes
- 4 slices back bacon
- 1 chorizo sausage
- ½ lb soft cheese
- 7 oz vegetable stock
- 1 large onion, peeled and diced

2 tablespoons Greek yogurt
1 tablespoon olive oil
1 tablespoon garlic puree
Salt and pepper to taste

Optional

3 tablespoons basil
3 tablespoons rosemary

Instructions

1. Add olive oil, onion and garlic into the Instant Pot. Set the Instant Pot to the "Sauté" function until the onions are soft and almost translucent.
2. Place the potatoes and thinly sliced sausages into the pot and stir. If needed add a little more of the olive oil.
3. Add the slices bacon chunks and the seasoning and let the pot simmer for a while.
4. Add the stock and set your Instant Pot to the "Soup" setting and set the timer for 10 minutes. Seal the lid and turn the valve to "Sealing."
5. Unlock the valve for pressure release once the timer goes off. Drain the remaining stock water before placing in a mixing bowl or large serving dish.
6. Add basil and rosemary. Mix in the Greek yogurt and soft cheese.
7. Serve and enjoy!

French Dip Sandwiches

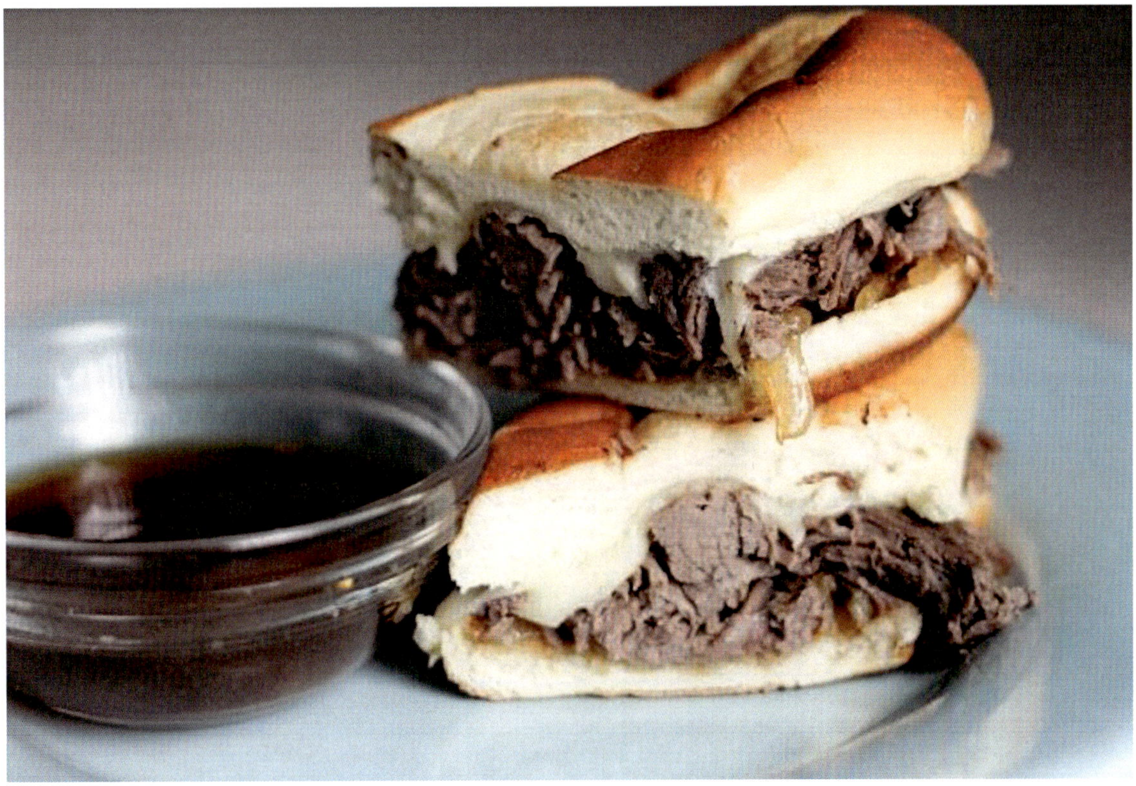

Prep Time: 15 minutes. Cook Time: 1 hour 40 minutes. Total Time: 1 hour 55 minutes.

This sandwiches that would normally take hours on end can, however, be enjoyed after only 2 hours with an Instant Pot. The tender beef roast chunks topped with melted cheese and covered with toasted garlic bread is sure to taste like it took you the whole day.

Servings: 6

Ingredients

2½ lb chuck roast
6 slices provolone cheese
6 soft sandwich rolls
14 oz can beef broth, low-sodium
½ cup red wine
1 onion, diced and thinly sliced
1 bay leaf, dried
3 tablespoon butter, melted
1 tablespoon vegetable oil
½ teaspoon garlic powder
¼ teaspoon garlic powder
Freshly ground pepper and kosher to taste

Instructions

1. Leave the chuck roast to rest for about 15 minutes at room temperature.
2. Add the vegetable oil in the Instant Pot and set it to "Sauté" function.
3. Season all sides of the chuck roast with ½ teaspoon garlic powder, salt and freshly ground paper.
4. Sear the chuck roast in the Instant Pot then set it aside.
5. Place the onions in the Instant Pot and sauté them until they start to soften and become translucent.
6. Pour the red wine into the Instant Pot and leave it to come to a boil and reduced by half. As the pot simmers use a wooden spoon to deglaze the bottom.
7. Add in the bay leaf and beef broth. Place the chuck roast back into the Instant Pot and close the lid.
8. Ensure the Pressure Release valve is positioned to "Sealing." Program the Instant Pot to "Meat/Stew" setting and set the cook time to 1 hour 40 minutes.
9. Allow Natural Release for about 25 minutes once the timer goes off then turn the Pressure Release Valve to "Venting" to release the excess steam.
10. Carefully open the lid and place the chuck roast on a serving plate and shred it to smaller pieces.
11. Mix together the ¼ teaspoon of garlic powder, the melted butter and a pinch of salt. Brush this mixture over the sandwich roll and toast them for at least 2-3 minutes, when they are golden brown.
12. Pile the shredded meat on the sandwich rolls the top with cheese. Place them in an oven to melt the cheese.
13. Garnish with freshly chopped parsley and serve.
14. Enjoy!

Stuffed Bell Peppers

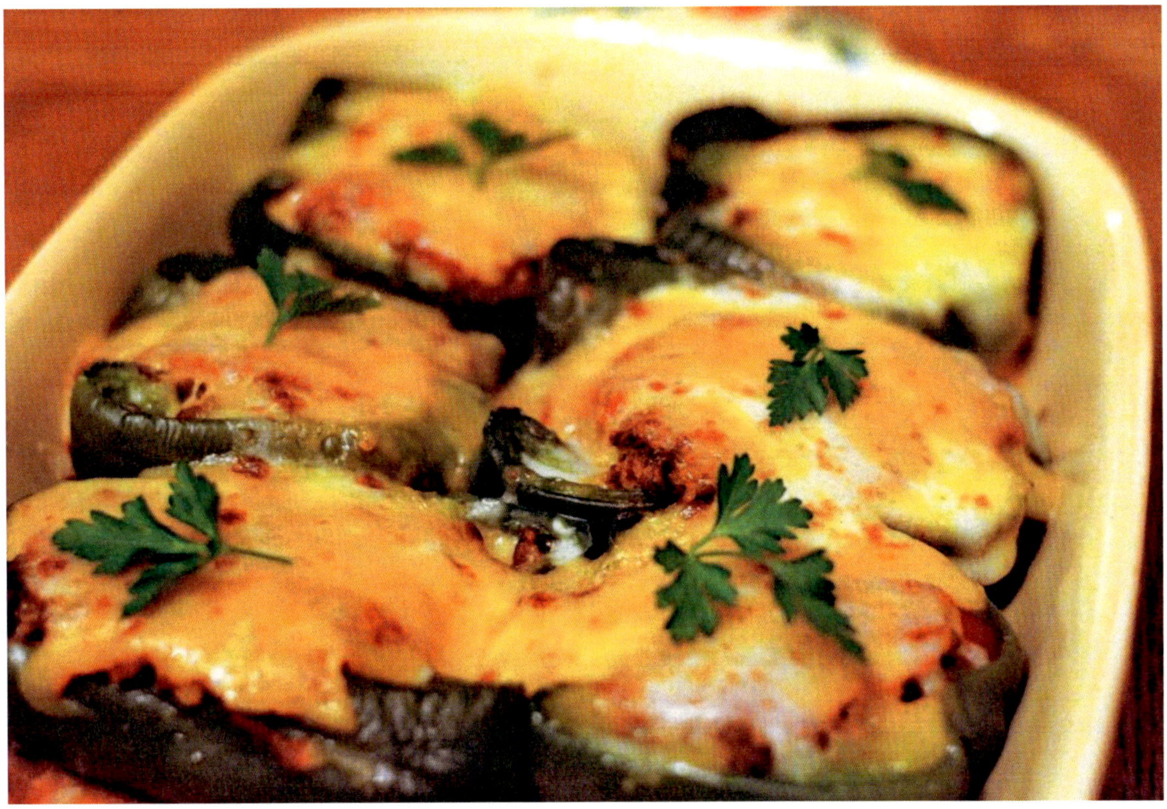

Prep Time: 10 minutes. Cook Time: 15 minutes. Total Time: 25 minutes.

Veggies make great appetizers and side dishes; the Instant Pot Stuffed Bell Peppers recipe is a delicious and healthy meal. To avoid the fat from the ground beef accumulating in the bell peppers poke a few holes at the bottom of the bell peppers before cooking.

Servings: 4

Ingredients

- 4 bell peppers
- 1 lb ground beef
- 1 cup brown rice, boiled
- 1 egg
- Mozzarella cheese, shredded
- 1 small onion, finely diced and sliced
- 15 oz can tomato sauce
- 1 onion, diced
- Dried parsley
- Garlic powder
- Oregano
- Salt and pepper, to taste

Instructions

1. Slice off the top of the bell peppers and hollow them. Dice the sliced pepper tops.
2. Mix the diced pepper tops, tomato, and onions with egg, ground beef, rice, some tomato sauce, and seasonings.
3. Fill the bell peppers with the combined mixture.
4. Pour 2/3 cups water and 2/3 tomato sauce into the Instant Pot. Place a trivet in the Pot and carefully put the stuffed bell peppers on the trivet. Pour any remaining tomato sauce on the bell peppers.
5. Seal the lid. Set the Instant Pot to "Manual" function and set the cook time for 15 minutes.
6. Allow Natural Pressure Release once the timer goes off. Carefully open the lid and sprinkle the mozzarella cheese on the pepper. Close the lid and let the cheese melt.
7. Place the stuffed bell peppers on a serving plate.
8. Enjoy!

Cabbage with Sausage

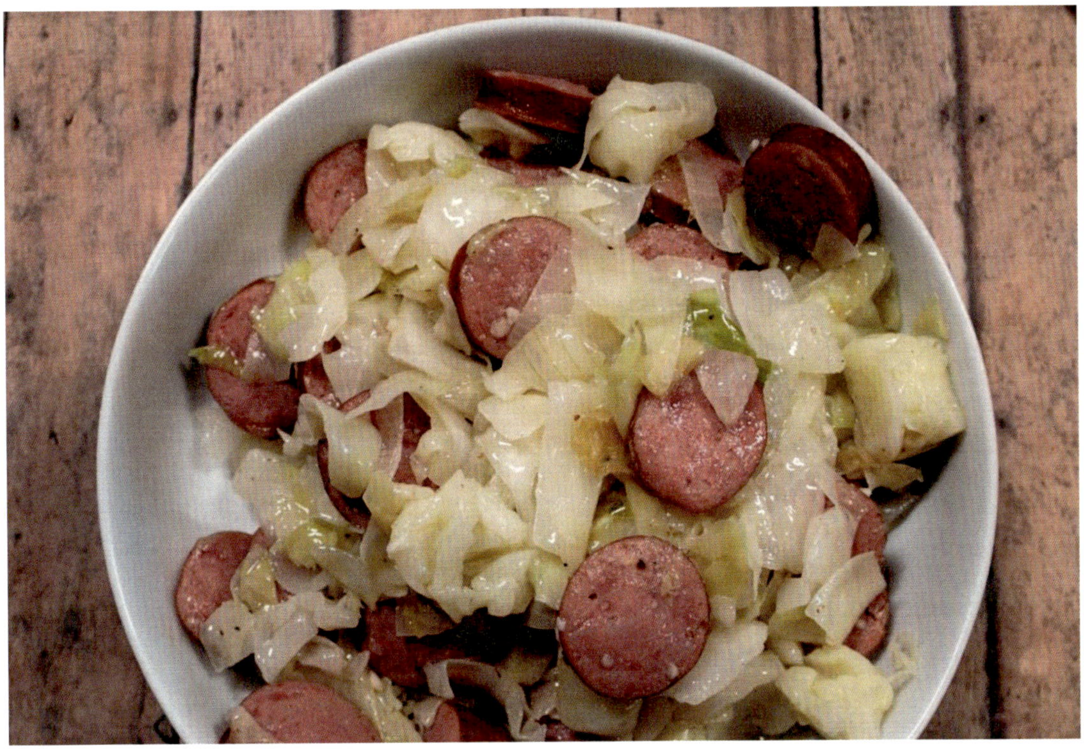

Prep Time: 3 minutes. Cook Time: 5 minutes. Total Time: 8 minutes.

You either love cabbage or hate it. Instant Pot veggies recipes are sure to change your mind. The recipe is filling you could actually eat it as a stand-alone meal.

Servings: 4-6

Ingredients

- 1 head cabbage, washed, cut and sliced
- 1 lb sausage (preference), sliced
- Olive oil
- 1 onion, finely diced
- 3 cloves garlic, minced
- 2 teaspoons Dijon mustard
- 2 teaspoons balsamic vinegar
- 2 teaspoons sugar
- Salt and pepper to taste

Instructions

1. Program the Instant Pot to "Sauté" function. Heat the olive oil then add the onions and sausages. Cook for 2-3 minutes until slightly browned.
2. Add the cabbage and all the other remaining ingredients in the Instant Pot. Cook for about 2 minutes until the cabbage softens.
3. Taste the cabbage and adjust the seasonings.
4. Serve and enjoy!

DESSERTS

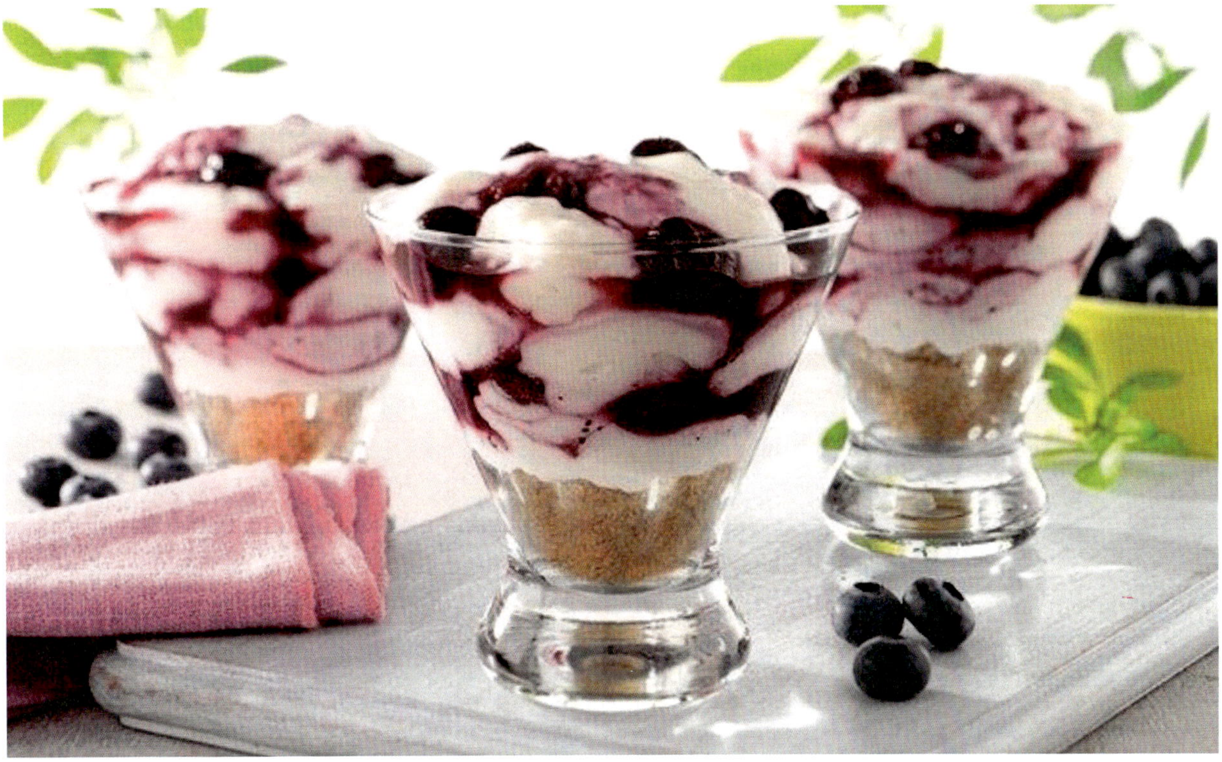

Baking and desserts aren't everyone's forte, and we get it. Cold or hot, desserts, in general, can make or break a meal. Much like the Instant Pot has made the culinary experience an easier feat for home-cooks, it's about to change your baking mistakes into sweet, decadent, savory or healthy memorable treats every time with minimal effort. With an Instant Pot make desserts in just half the usual required time making it the must-have kitchen accessory, not even the oven can match up to it. Finish your every meal in style with these no-fuss, top-rated and delicious homemade desserts recipes that are sure to please. You will always have these luscious dessert options for your sweet tooth.

Apple Crisp

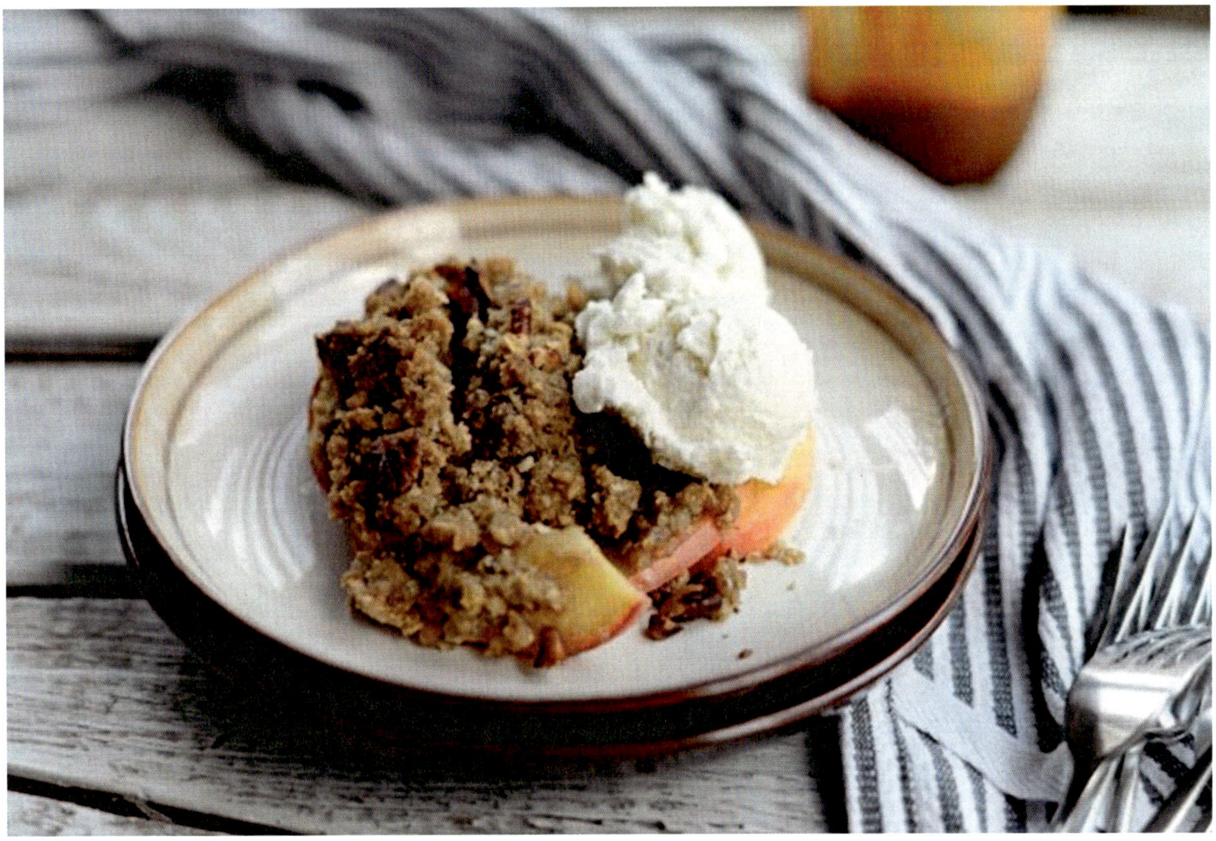

Prep Time: 5 minutes. Cook Time: 8 minutes. Total Time: 13 minutes.

Take full advantage of every apple season by baking with apples. The Instant Pot Apple Crisp is a great apple dessert recipe with just the right amount of sweetness and simple, wholesome ingredients that are easily available. With a nice crispy top, the Instant Pot Apple crisp is just perfection in every sense.

Servings: 3-4

Ingredients

- 5 medium apples, peeled and roughly chopped
- ¼ cup brown sugar
- ¼ cup flour
- ¾ cup old-fashioned rolled oats
- ½ cup water
- 4 tablespoons butter
- 1 tablespoon maple syrup
- 2 teaspoon cinnamon
- ½ teaspoon nutmeg
- ½ teaspoon salt

Toppings (Optional)

Vanilla ice cream

Instructions

1. Place the apples in the Instant Pot then sprinkle with nutmeg and cinnamon. Top the apples with maple syrup and pour in water.
2. Melt the butter. Then make a mixture of the melted butter, flour, oats, salt and brown sugar in a small bowl. Add this mixture to the Instant Pot.
3. Seal the lid and program the Instant Pot to "Manual" setting the cook on "High Pressure" for 8 minutes.
4. Once the timer goes off, allow Natural Pressure Release. Let the sauce sit for a while for it to thicken.
5. Top with vanilla ice cream and serve warm.
6. Enjoy!

Mini-Lemon Cheesecakes

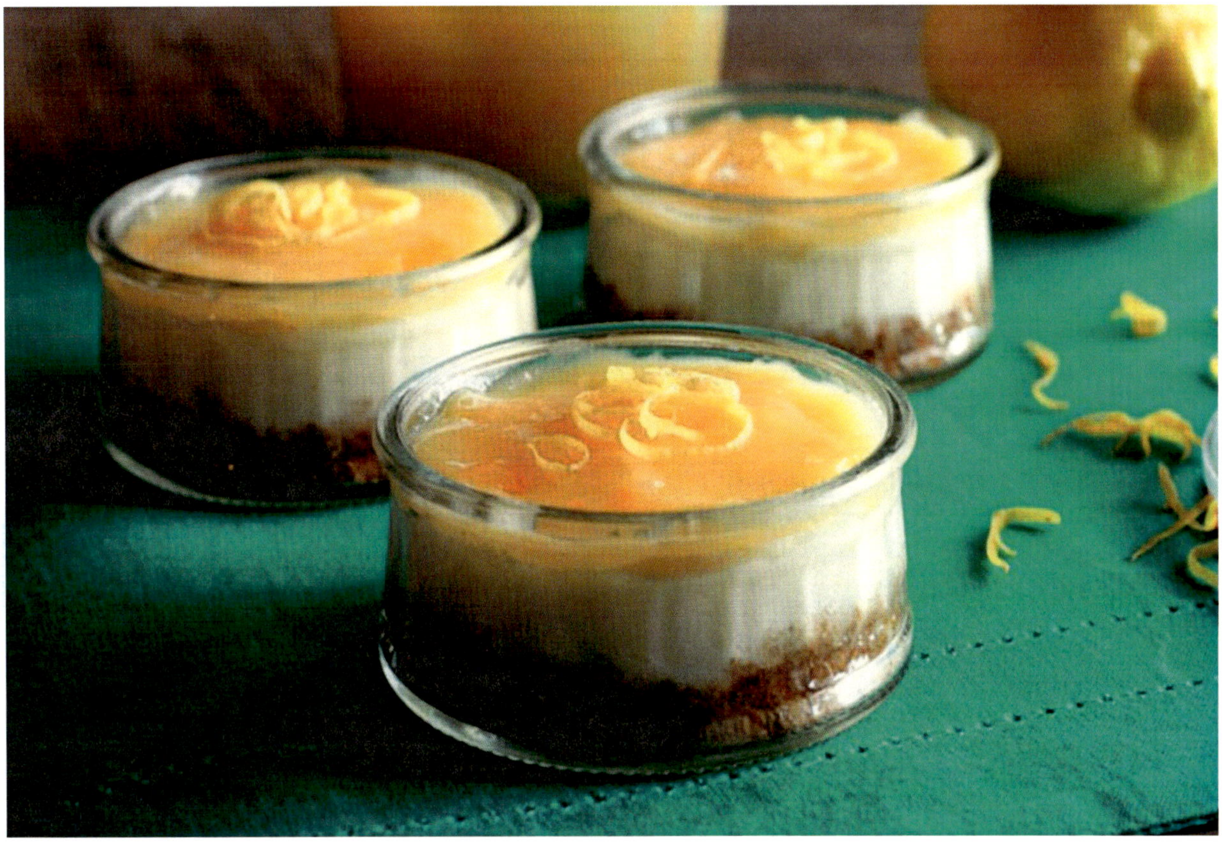

Prep Time: 10 minutes. Cook Time: 8 minutes. Total Time: 18 minutes.

For a pop of citrus flavor try out the Instant Pot crust-less mini cheesecake recipe. The low-carb cheesecake has a tasty surprise lemon curd right in the middle. You can easily get all the ingredients on your weekly grocery run, this way you have a dessert to top off dinner even on a school night. Mini-Lemon Cheesecakes are a great and healthy recipe for the kids. Make it ahead and set aside to cool in the refrigerator for later.

Servings: 6

Ingredients

- 16 oz cream cheese, room temp
- ½ cup sour cream, room temp
- ½ cup sugar
- 1½ cups water
- 3 eggs
- 1 jar lemon curd
- 1 lemon zest
- 1 tablespoon lemon juice
- 1 teaspoon flour
- ½ teaspoon vanilla
- 6 mason jars (1/2 pint)

Optional

Raspberries
Sliced lemon

Instructions

1. Add cream cheese, flour, and sugar in a large mixing bowl then stir the ingredients into a smooth, creamy mixture with no lumps.
2. Add the sour cream, lemon zest, and lemon juice into the mixture and continue stirring. Beat one egg at a time into the mixture and lightly stir the mixture.
3. Fill ¼ of all the mason jars with the cheesecake batter. Gently drop a tablespoon of the lemon curd on top of the batter before filling an additional ¼ of the jars with the remaining cheesecake batter. Loosely cover the jars with foil.
4. Add 1½ cups of water into the Instant Pot and place the trivet into the pot. Carefully arrange the fitting jars on the steam rack trivet and stack the remaining jars on top of the others.
5. Seal the lid. Set the Instant Pot at "Manual" setting and cook on "High Pressure" for 8 minutes.
6. Allow Natural Pressure Release for about 15 minutes once the timer goes off. Carefully remove the jars and allow them to cool to room temperature before refrigerating.
7. When ready to serve garnish with more lemon curd and raspberries or lemon slice.
8. Enjoy!

Apple Bread with Salted Caramel Icing

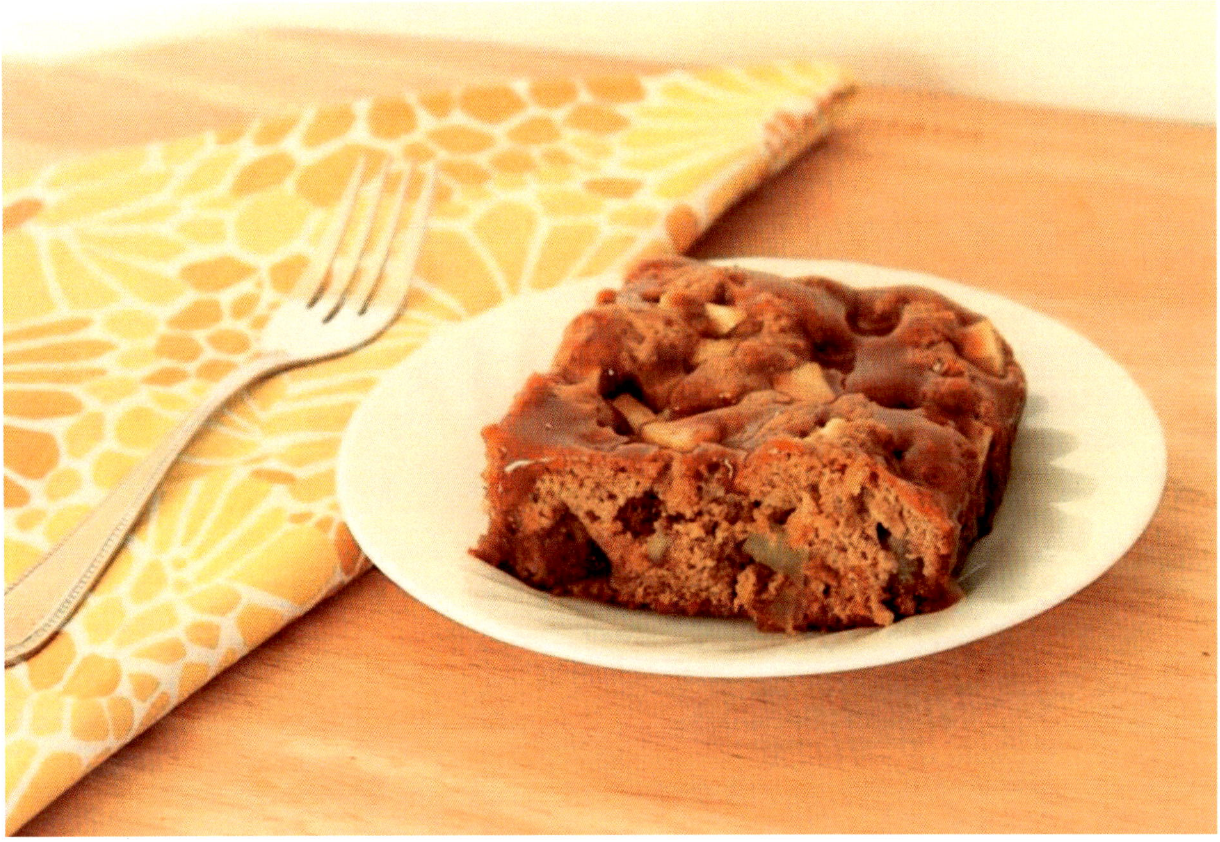

Prep Time: 10 minutes. Cook Time: 1 hour 10 minutes. Total Time: 1 hour 20 minutes.

Everyone knows fall season is all about the falling leaves, but it's also time to break out those delicious apple recipes. Apple bread is one of those recipes, the moist bread topped off with salted caramel icing makes an unforgettable dessert option.

Servings: 6-8.

Ingredients

3 cups apples; peeled, cored and cut it cubes
2 cups flour
1 stick butter
1 cup sugar
2 eggs
1 teaspoon apple pie spice
1 teaspoon baking powder
1 teaspoon vanilla.

Toppings

2 cups powdered sugar

2 cups brown sugar
1 cup heavy cream
1 stick butter

Instructions

Apple bread

1. Add butter, eggs, sugar, apple pie spice into the mixer and cream together the ingredients into a smooth mixture. Then stir in the apples.
2. Mix flour and baking powder in another mixing bowl and add this flour mixture to the wet mix.
3. Add 1 cup of water in the Instant Pot and place the steam rack into the pot. Add the batter into a 7" Springform pan and place on the steam rack.
4. Seal the lid. Program the Instant Pot to "Manual" setting and cook at "High Pressure" for 70 minutes.
5. Allow a Quick Pressure Release once the timer goes off. Open the lid and carefully remove the cake.

Icing

6. Melt the butter before adding the brown sugar. Let the mixture to come to a boil.
7. Continue cooking for an additional 3 minutes until the sugar is melted. Before stirring in the heavy cream and continue cooking for about 2-3 minutes until the mixture slightly thickens.
8. Remove the mixture from the heat and cool.
9. Top with powdered sugar and whisk until smooth and creamy.
10. Top the apple bread with icing serve and enjoy.

Sticky Toffee Pudding

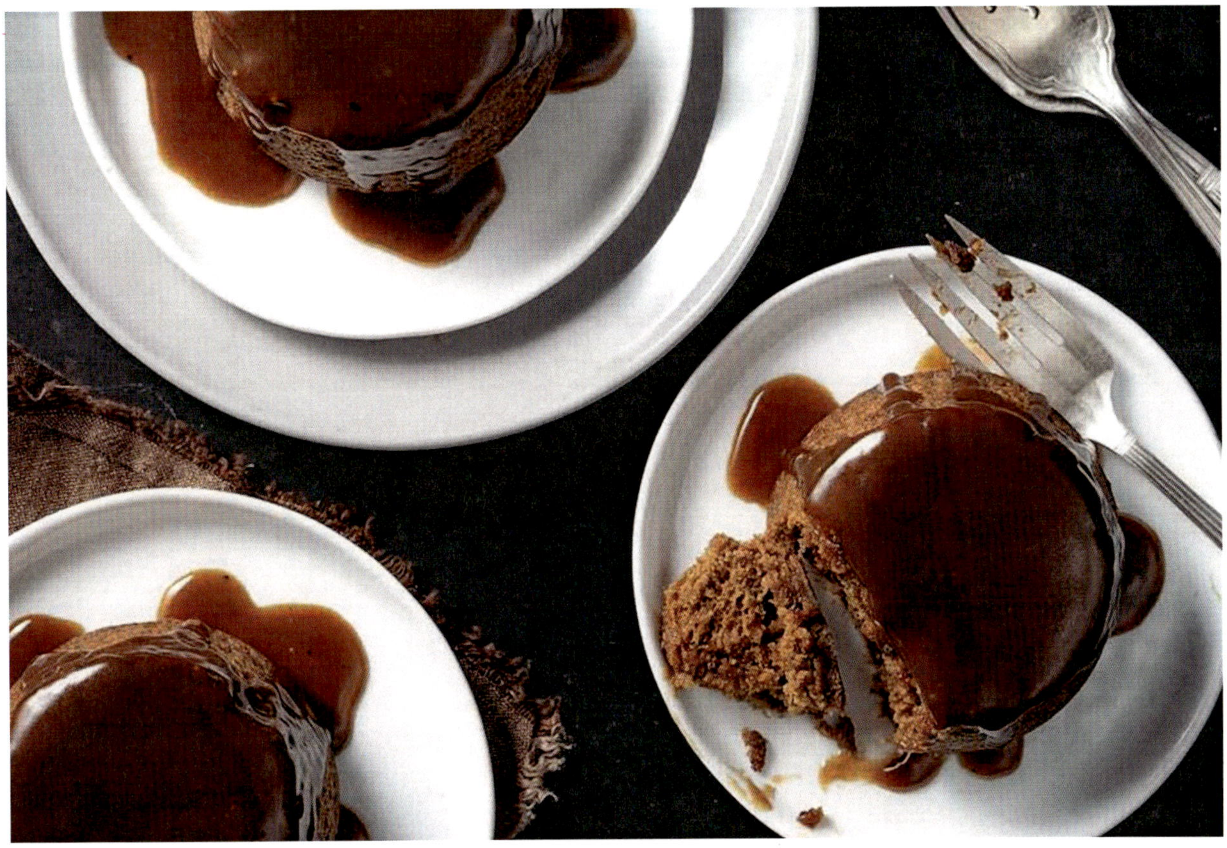

Prep Time: 30 minutes. Cook Time: 20 minutes. Total Time: 50 minutes.

If you prefer sweet, warm, decadent desserts, then the Sticky Toffee Pudding is the perfect warm pudding. Traditionally made in an oven, the brown sugar, dates and molasses filled dense pudding can easily be made in the Instant Pot. The rich caramel sauce glaze works well with the pudding. The best part is the pudding is freezer-friendly, so you can preserve the leftover for a delightful dessert on another night.

Servings: 8

Ingredients

Pudding

1¼ cups all-purpose flour
¾ cup water, boiling
1 egg
1½ cups dates, finely chopped
¾ cup brown sugar
¼ cup blackstrap molasses
1/3 cup unsalted butter, room temp
1 teaspoon baking powder
1 teaspoon vanilla extract
¼ teaspoon salt

Caramel sauce

¼ cup unsalted butter
1/3 cup whipping cream
2/3 cup dark brown sugar
1 teaspoon vanilla extract

Instructions

Pudding

1. Grease 8 ramekins with butter and set them aside.
2. Add the boiling water, dates and molasses in one mixing bowl. Combine the ingredients and let the mixture cool.
3. Add salt, baking powder and flour in another bowl and mix them.
4. Use a mixer to cream the butter and brown sugar until fluffy. Beat in the vanilla extract and egg into the mixture.
5. One after the other, add the other mixtures into the large mixing bowl with the butter and brown sugar mixture. Thoroughly beat the mixture after each addition.
6. Equally, divide the smooth batter into the 8 greased ramekins.
7. Carefully cover and seal each ramekin with a buttered foil.
8. Pour 2 cups of water into the Instant Pot and place the trivet into the pot. Carefully stack the ramekins on the trivet and seal the lid.
9. Program the Instant Pot to "Manual" setting, cook at "High Pressure" for a couple of minutes and adjust to "Medium Low" then cook for 20 minutes.
10. Do a Quick Pressure Release once the timer goes off and open the lid. Carefully remove the ramekins and remove the foil.

Caramel Sauce

11. Start working on the caramel sauce while the puddings are cooking.
12. In a saucepan combine whipping cream, butter, vanilla and brown sugar.
13. Bring the mixture to a boil and cook for a few more minutes until the sugar dissolves.
14. Reduce the heat and let the sauce simmer for an additional 5 minutes.
15. Remove from heat; your sauce should be smooth and slightly thicken.
16. Pour the caramel over the puddings
17. Serve your sticky toffee pudding warm and enjoy.

Molten Chocolate Lava Cake

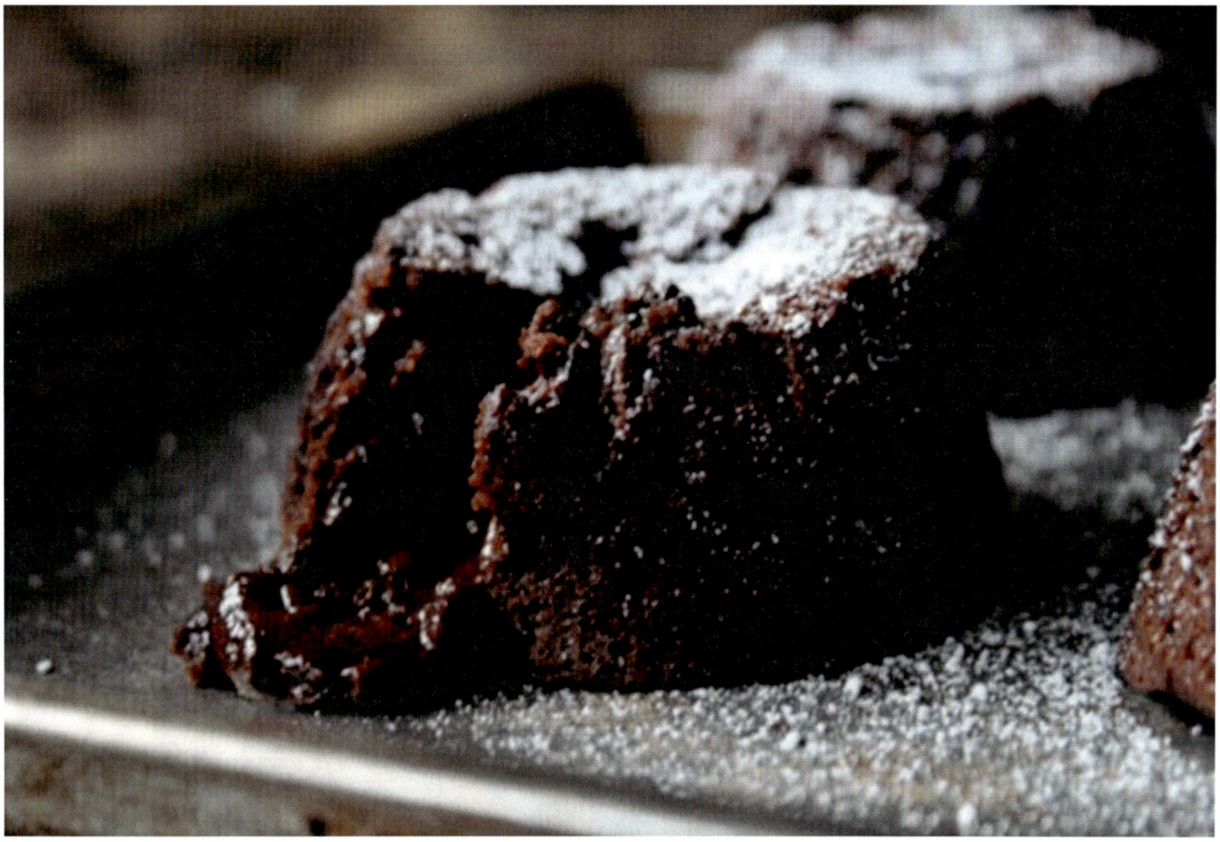

Prep Time: 10 minutes. **Cook Time: 9 minutes.** **Total Time: 19 minutes.**

The hint of coffee and a gooey chocolate center makes the Instant Pot Molten Chocolate Lava Cake a wonderfully decadent chocolate treat. With a short prep time and an even shorter ingredients list, this Instant Pot dessert is quick and easy to make. There is no need for an oven to make a delicious and decadent dessert anymore.

Servings: 4

Ingredients

- 6 tablespoons all-purpose flour
- 1 cup confectioners' sugar
- 4 oz semisweet chocolate, chopped
- 1 stick (1/2 cup) butter, cut into pieces
- 2 eggs
- 2 egg yolks
- 1 tablespoon granulated sugar
- 1 teaspoon vanilla extract
- 1 teaspoon instant coffee granules
- ¼ teaspoon salt

Instructions

1. Generously grease 4 ramekins and coat them with sugar.
2. Melt the chocolate and butter in the microwave until the combination is smooth and all melted.
3. Place the chocolate and butter melted mixture in a small mixing bowl and stir in confectioner's sugar.
4. Whisk in the eggs and yolks and top with vanilla and coffee and stir the mixture.
5. Finally, add in the flour and salt and stir until the mixture is smooth and creamy.
6. Equally, pour the batter into the 4 ramekins.
7. Pour 2 cups of water into the Instant Pot and Place a steam rack into the pot. Carefully place the ramekins on the steam rack, stack the ramekins if they don't all fit.
8. Close the lid and ensure that the Steam Release Valve is in "Sealing" position.
9. Program the Instant pot to "Manual" setting and cook at "High Pressure" for 9 minutes.
10. Do a Quick Pressure Release once the timer goes off and carefully open the lid. Gently remove the ramekins and dab off condensation.
11. Dust the molten chocolate lava cakes with powdered sugar and serve them when they are still warm.
12. Enjoy!

Instant Pot Flan

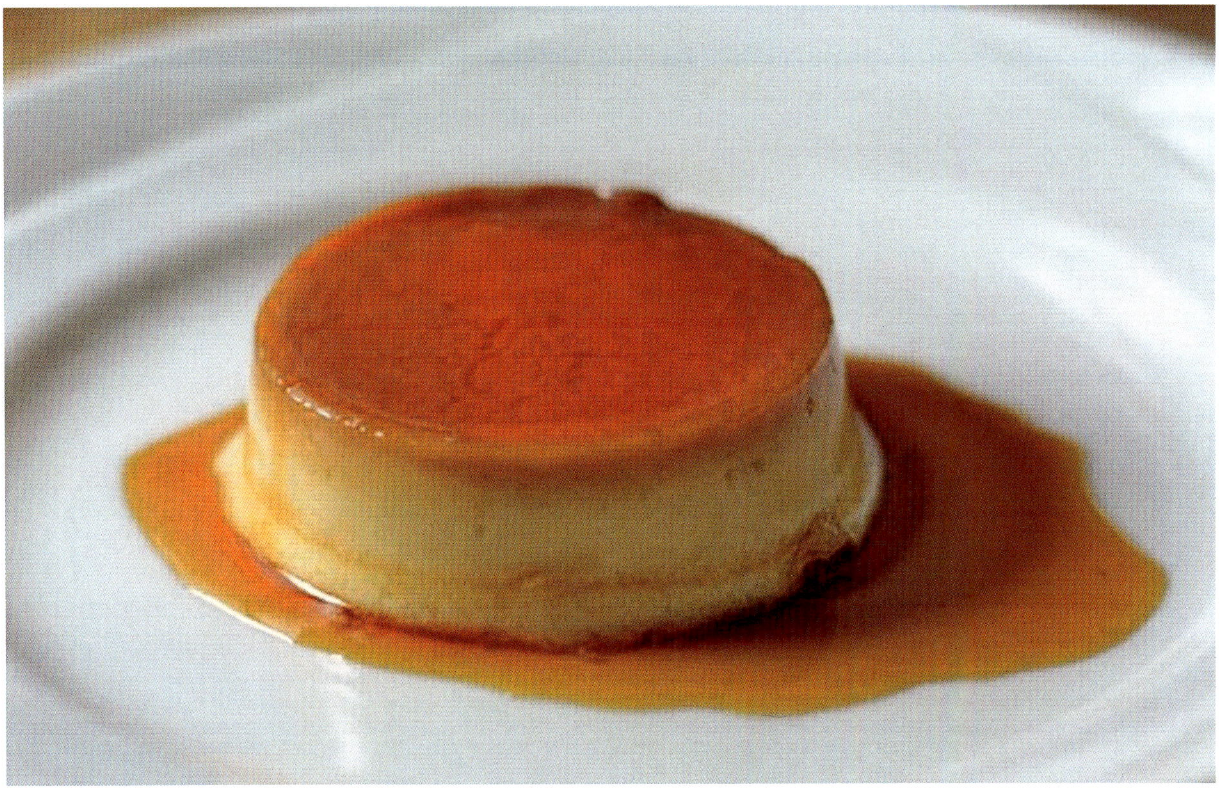

Prep Time: 25 minutes. Cook Time: 9 minutes. Total Time: 34 minutes.

Whether you want to call it a caramel pudding, crème caramel or caramel custard, this is one of those silky-smooth Instant Pot dessert recipes you need to try out. You will fall in love over and over with its silky-smooth texture, the sweet aromas and flavors of the caramel as it slowly and delicately melts in your mouth. Amaze your dinner party guests with this quick and easy to make Instant Pot dessert recipe.

Servings: 6

Ingredients

Caramel

½ cup white sugar
2 tablespoons water

Flan

3 extra large eggs, beaten lightly
¼ cup sugar
1 cup milk (2%)
1 cup heavy cream
1 pinch salt
2 teaspoons vanilla extract

Instructions

1. To make caramel heat water and sugar in a saucepan over Medium-High heat. Stir the mixture occasionally until it turns to a dark golden-brown color. Equally divide the caramel in 6, ramekins and leave to cool.
2. Pour milk and the heavy cream in a medium pot and heat. Once this mixture is hot, add in vanilla extract, sugar and sea salt and stir until till the sugar dissolves fully.
3. In another medium bowl, lightly beat the eggs. Slowly pour in little portions of the milk mixture to bring up the eggs' temperature. Whisk continuously until you've poured in all the milk mixture.
4. Top the caramel-filled ramekins with this mixture. Pour in the mixture through a strainer. Use a blowtorch or a spoon to remove any bubbles. Tightly cover ramekins with aluminum foil pieces.
5. Pour ½ cup of water into the Instant Pot and place the steam rack in the pot. Place the ramekins on the steam rack and seal the lid. Set the Instant Pot to cook at "High Pressure" for 9 minutes.
6. Allow Natural Pressure Release and carefully open the lid and gently remove the ramekins.
7. Set the flans to cool before refrigerating them overnight (or at least 4 hours) to firm up before serving.
8. Carefully invert the ramekins on a serving plate to remove the flans.
9. Serve cold and enjoy!

Fudgy Brownie Sundaes

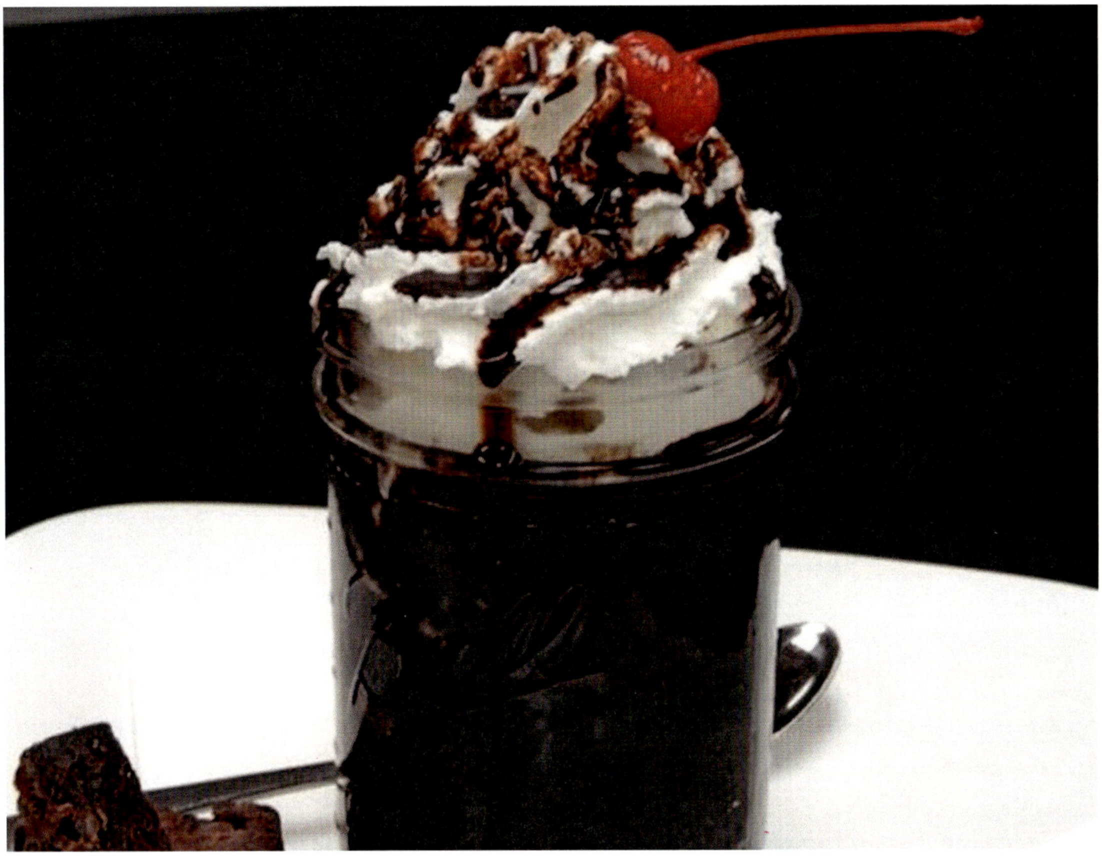

Prep Time: 15 minutes. Cook Time: 20 minutes. Total Time: 35 minutes.

These delicious individual-sized desserts are sure to satisfy your sweet tooth any time. The Instant Pot Fudgy Brownie Sundaes are quick and easy to make. That's why they are always a welcomed treat.

Servings: 7.

Ingredients

2/3 cup all-purpose flour
Vanilla ice cream
1 stick butter, unsalted
2 eggs, room temp
4 oz bittersweet chocolate, chopped
¾ cup sugar
½ teaspoon vanilla extract
¼ teaspoon instant coffee granules
½ teaspoon salt
1 package crème de menthe candies, roughly chopped (optional)

Toppings (Optional)

Chocolate sauce

Chocolate Shavings
Nuts
Berries

Instructions

1. Lightly grease 7 half-pint mason jars with cooking spray and set them aside.
2. Add instant coffee granules, salt, and flour in a bowl and combine them into a mixture.
3. In a small bowl melt the chocolate and butter in the microwave for 30 seconds. Halfway through stir the mixture.
4. Whisk in sugar then eggs and vanilla into chocolate and butter mixture until the mixture is smooth.
5. Finally, stir in the flour mixture and the crème menthe candies (optional).
6. Equally, divide the batter into the greased mason jars and cover each jar with aluminum foil.
7. Pour 1 cup of water into the Instant Pot and place a trivet in the Instant Pot.
8. Carefully place the mason jars in the Instant Pot and close the lid. Ensure the Steam Release Handle is in the "Sealing" Position.
9. Program the Instant to cook on "Manual" setting for 20 minutes. Once the timer goes off, do a Quick Pressure Release and carefully open the lid.
10. Remove the mason jars and carefully dab any condensation on the surface and allow the brownies to cool.
11. Top with a scoop of vanilla ice cream and garnish with your favorite toppings.
12. Serve and enjoy!

Banoffee Pie

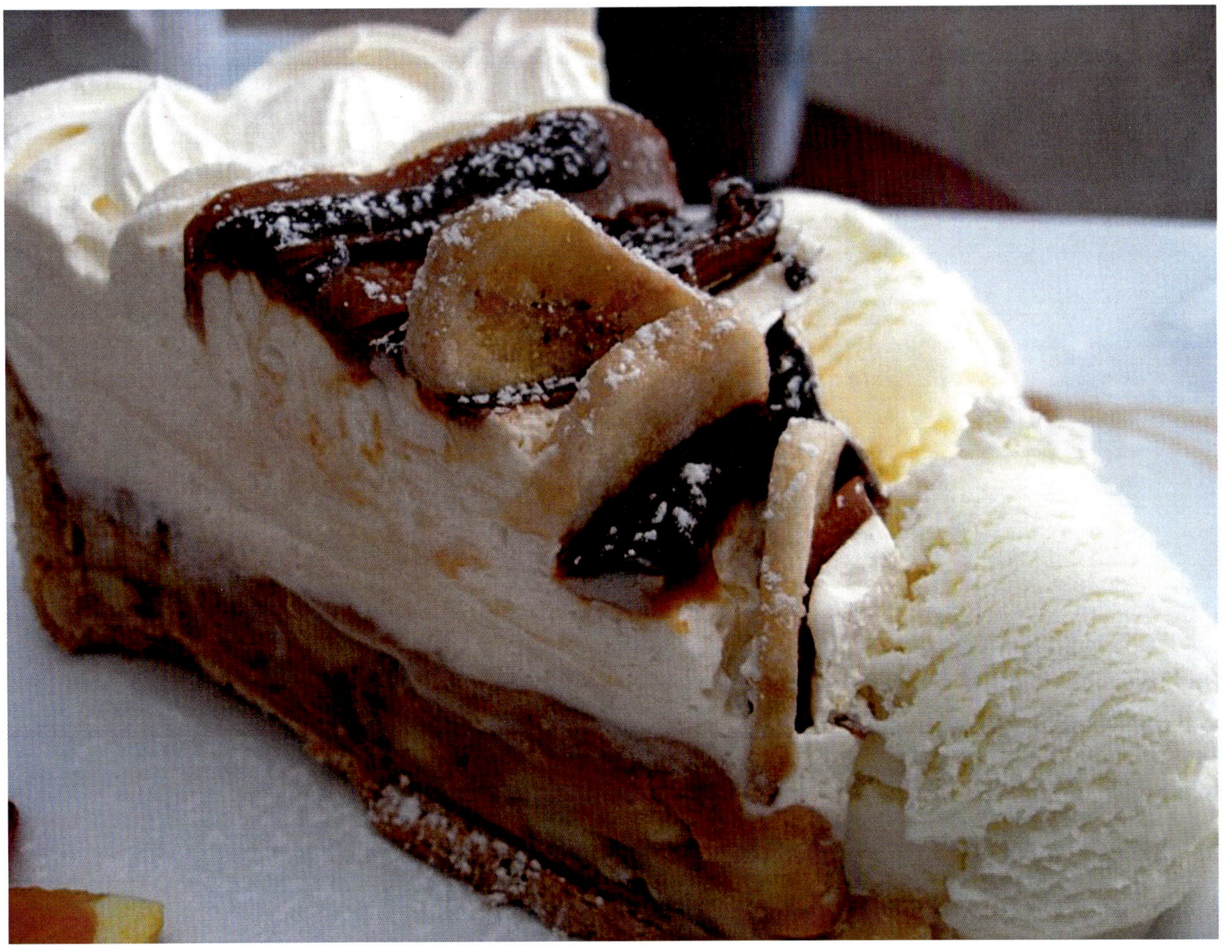

Prep Time: 15 minutes. Cook Time: 35 minutes. Total Time: 50 minutes.

Quite an odd name! The Banoffee (banana and toffee) pie is yet another heavenly dessert you can make in the comfort of your home courtesy of the Instant Pot. As far as Instant Pot dessert recipes go this banana filled, toffee sauce and cheesecake-like dessert is a must-try.

Servings: 8

Ingredients

3 bananas
1 can condensed milk
10 oz. Greek Yogurt
1 stick butter
½ lb Digestive biscuits
½ teaspoon vanilla essence

Optional

Caramel sauce

Instructions

1. Remove labels from the condensed milk can and lay it on its side in the Instant Pot. Pour water into the Instant Pot until the condensed milk can is submerged.
2. Cover the lid and ensure the Steam Releasing valve is set to "Sealing" position. Program the Instant to cook on "Manual" setting for 35 minutes.
3. While the milk cooks, crush the digestive biscuits and melt the stick of butter in a saucepan. Add the crushed biscuits into the melted butter and stir to make a mixture. Add the mixture to a baking tin compact it down. Then place the baking tin in the fridge and allow the compacted mixture to cool and set into a crust.
4. Once the timer goes off, do a Quick Pressure Release, carefully open the lid and remove the condensed milk can. Set it aside and allow it to cool for half an hour.
5. Place the contents of the condensed milk can in a mixing bowl. Slice the bananas and add the pieces in the mixing bowl and mix well.
6. Remove the crust from fridge and pour the contents of the mixing bowl over the crust in the baking tin.
7. Add the vanilla essence to the yogurt, mix and top the banoffee pie. Lastly, drizzle with caramel sauce and serve.
8. Enjoy!

Rice Pudding

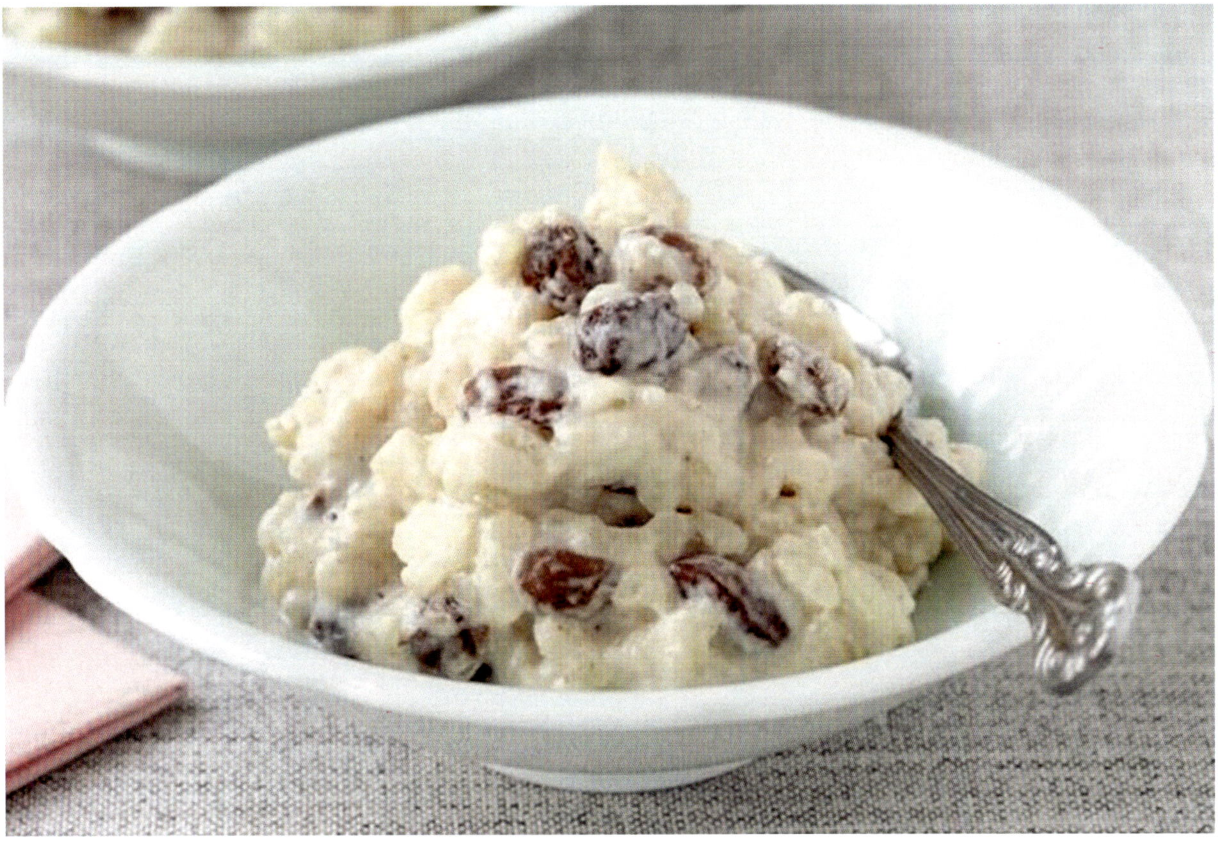

Prep Time: 10 minutes. Cook Time: 3 minutes. Total Time: 13 minutes.

Rice pudding is a comfort food on its own right. With an Instant Pot, you can make the creamy and delicious old-fashioned rice pudding much easier and quicker. Arborio rice makes an even creamier rice pudding without the hassle of adding any cream. Don't worry; you can still use any other type of rice without causing any significant changes to the recipe, all you need to do is adjust the cooking time.

Servings: 8.

Ingredients

- 1 cup Arborio rice
- 2 eggs
- 2 cups whole milk, divided
- 1½ cups water
- ½ cup sugar
- ¾ raisins
- ½ teaspoon vanilla extract
- ¼ teaspoon salt

Instructions

1. Add water, salt, and rice in the Instant Pot. Close the lid. Select the "Manual" setting and at High Pressure for 3 minutes. Allow Natural Pressure Release

for about 10 minutes once the timer goes off. After 10 minutes do a Quick Pressure Release and carefully open the lid.

2. Pour 1½ cups of milk over the cooked rice and stir thoroughly.
3. Whisk eggs, vanilla extract and the remaining ½ cup of milk in a small mixing bowl. Pour this mixture into the Instant Pot through a fine mesh strainer. Program the Instant Pot to the "Sauté" function stir the pot until the starts to simmer and turn off the Instant Pot.
4. Stir in the raisins and set aside your rice pudding. The pudding thickens as it cools but you can either serve it warm or cold.
5. Top with whipped cream and sprinkle nutmeg or cinnamon.
6. Serve and enjoy!

Chocolate Mousse

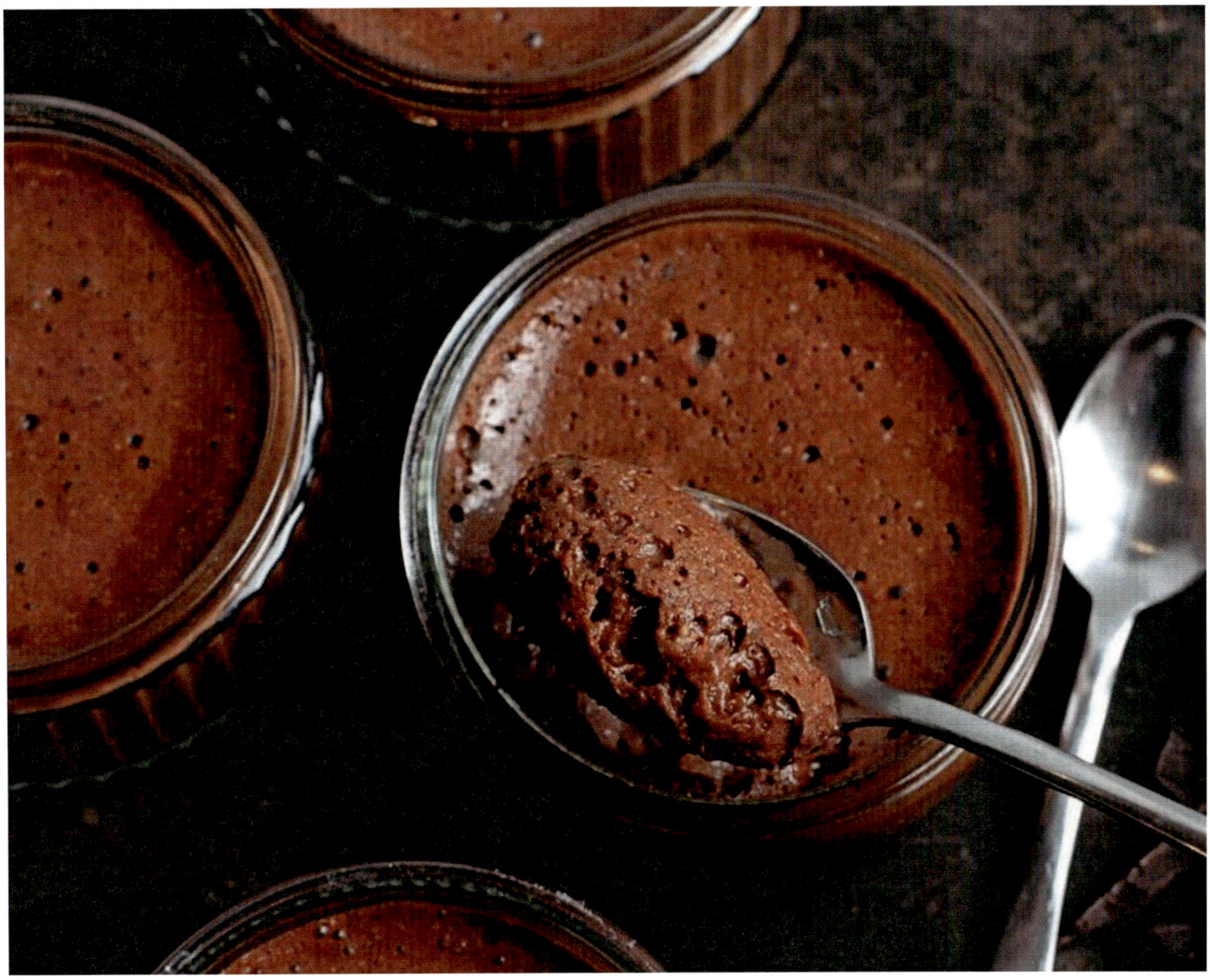

Prep Time: 15 minutes. Cook Time: 6 minutes. Total Time: 21 minutes.

Whether you are watching your carb intake or not, you are going to enjoy this tasty make-ahead low carb dessert. The rich, creamy, chocolatey treat that is the Instant Pot Chocolate Mousse is great for your health and your sweet tooth.

Servings: 5.

Ingredients

- 4 egg yolks
- 1 cup whipping cream
- ½ cup almond milk
- ½ cup swerve
- ¼ cup cacao
- ¼ cup water
- ½ teaspoon vanilla
- ½ teaspoon sea salt

Instructions

1. Beat the yolks in mixing bowl and set them aside.
2. Add water, swerve and cacao in a saucepan and heat the mixture over Medium-Heat. Keep stirring the mixture until the cacao is well combined and the sugar melts.
3. Then add almond milk and cream to the saucepan and continue to whisk until the mixture combines. Turn off the heat before the mixture comes to a boil.
4. Take the pan off the heat then mix in the salt and vanilla.
5. Slowly pour the warm chocolatey mixture into the bowl with the beaten yolks while whisking to combine into a smooth mixture.
6. Equally, pour the incorporated mixture into 5 ramekins or mason jars.
7. Add 1½ cups of water into the Instant Pot and place a trivet in the Pot. Carefully place the ramekins or mason jars on the trivet and close the lid.
8. Ensure the Steam Release Knob is on "Sealing" position and program the Instant Pot to cook on "Manual" setting for 6 minutes.
9. Do a Quick Pressure Release once the timer goes off and carefully open the lid. Take out the ramekins or jars and let them cool before refrigerating for at least 4-6 hours.
10. Serve and enjoy!

Baked Apples

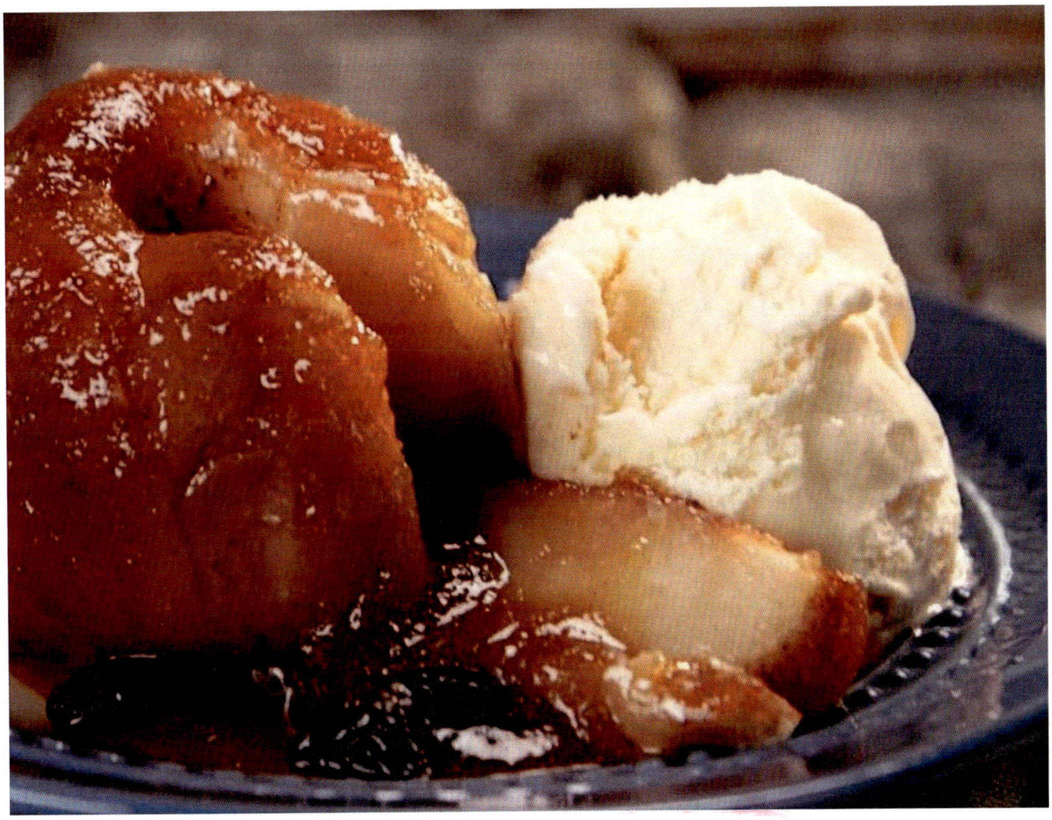

Prep Time: 2 minutes. Cook Time: 6 minutes. Total Time: 8 minutes.

Have you ever craved something healthy and sweet, but you were too lazy to prep and cook? In less than 10 minutes you could be indulging in a warm, fragrant bowl of baked apples. The Instant Pot Baked Apple recipe is the fastest and easiest way to make baked apples, and they are tasty.

Servings: 6

Ingredients

6 apples
½ cup sugar
1 cup apple juice
2 tablespoons cinnamon

Instructions

1. Core the apples and place them in the Instant Pot.
2. Pour the apple juice into the pot. Generously sprinkle the apples with sugar and cinnamon.
3. Seal the lid. Set the Instant Pot to cook on "Low Pressure" for about 6 minutes. You can either allow Natural Release or do a Quick Release once the cook time lapses.
4. Serve hot topped with either or both ice cream and whipped cream.

Tapioca Pudding

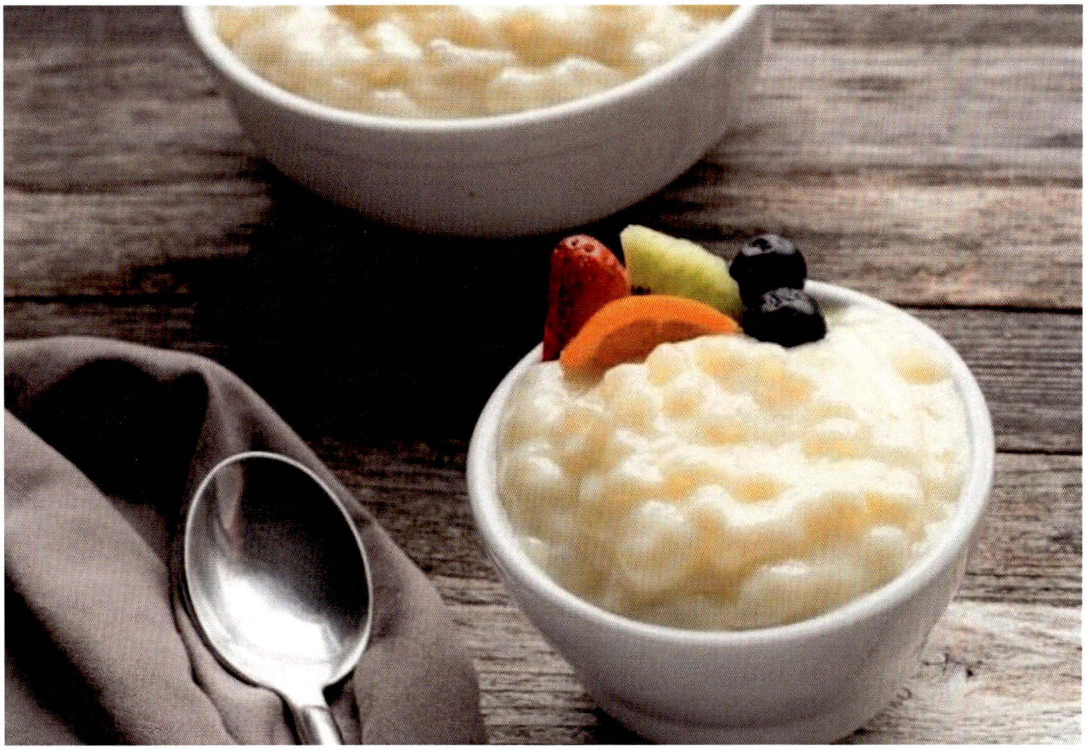

Prep Time: 5 minutes. Cook Time: 10 minutes. Total Time: 15 minutes.

If you grew up on Tapioca, then you know it tastes great cold or warm. This Tapioca Pudding recipe is a simple dessert idea and a kid's favorite because all you really need is milk.

Servings: 5

Ingredients

3 tablespoons instant tapioca
2 ¾ cups milk
1 egg
1/3 cup sugar
1 teaspoon vanilla

Instructions

1. Place 2 cups of water into the Instant Pot and put a steam rack in the pot.
2. Add the tapioca, milk, sugar, and vanilla in an inner pot then stir to combine the ingredients. Whisk in the egg. Cover the inner pot with a foil.
3. Place the inner pot on the steam rack and close the lid. Ensure the Steam Valve is set to "Sealing." Program the Instant Pot to "Manual" and cook at "High Pressure" for 10 minutes.
4. Once the Instant Pot beeps do a Quick Release, it might be messy because the steam might contain a bit of milk. Alternatively, you can allow Natural Release for about 5 minutes.

5. Carefully open the lid and remove the inner pot. Set it aside to cool.
6. Stir and put back the foil and refrigerate overnight.
7. Serve and enjoy!

Caramel Pot de Crème

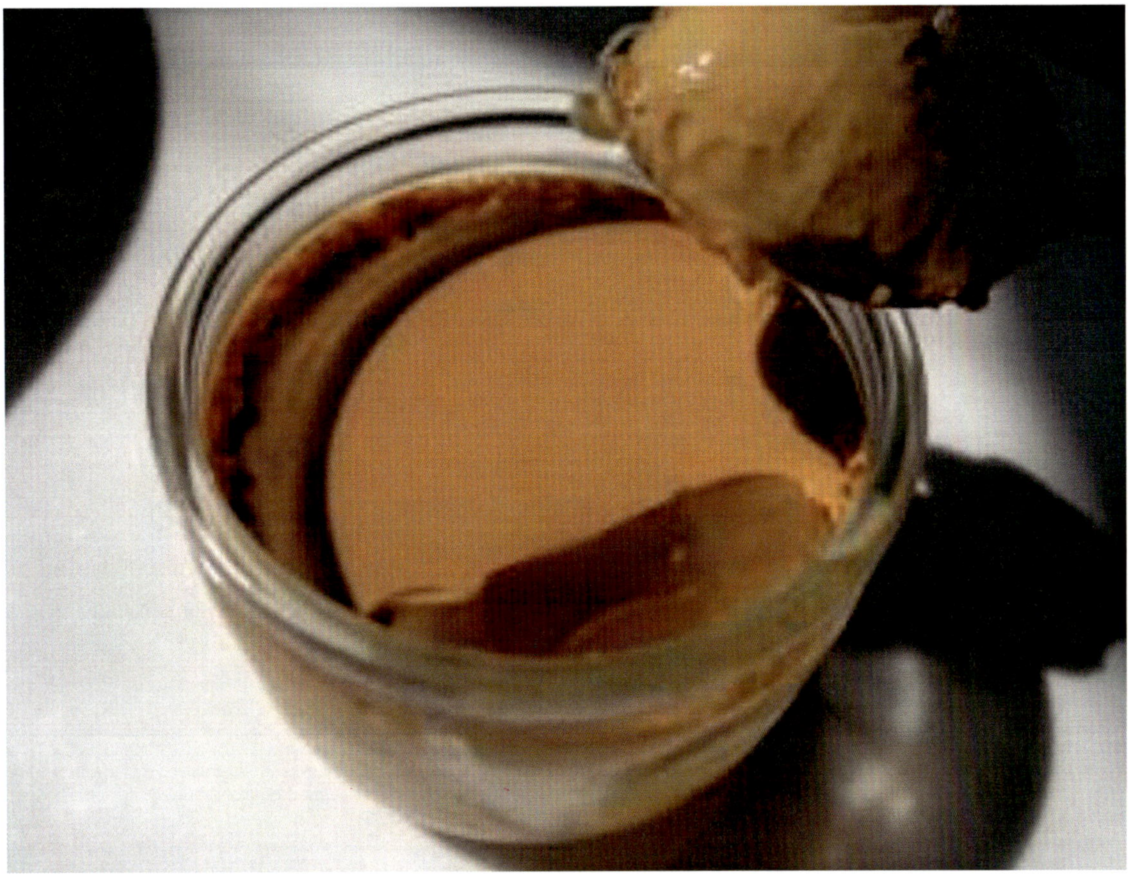

Prep Time: 10 minutes. Cook Time: 10 minutes. Total Time: 20 minutes.

If you try this recipe, then be aware that you will want to make these luscious, and decadent Caramel Pot de Crèmes over and over. They are tasty, and you might just dive in before they are ready to serve. The Caramel Pot de Crèmes are true to the phrase goodness in every bite.

Servings: 4

Ingredients

3 large egg yolks
1 cup heavy whipping cream
1/3 cup granulated sugar
¼ cup water
½ teaspoon vanilla extract

Optional

Sea salt

Instructions

1. In a small mixing bowl whisk, the egg yolks then set them aside.

2. In a saucepan add water and sugar and stir. Heat the mixture until it boils.
3. Lower the heat to Medium-High and allow the sugar mixture to continue boiling until it turns brown.
4. Reduce the heat to Medium-Low then whisk in the whipping cream slowly until it dissolves fully.
5. First, add a tablespoon of the caramel and whipping cream mixture to the egg yolks and mix it into a mixture. Continue adding the remaining mixture into the egg yolks and whisk until all the ingredients are fully incorporated.
6. Add vanilla to the mixture and continue stirring. Equally, divide the mixture into 4 mason jars or ramekins.
7. Pour 1½ cups of water into the Instant Pot and Place a trivet in the pot. Carefully place the mason jars or ramekins on the trivet and seal the lid.
8. Program the Instant to "Manual" setting and cook at "High Pressure" for 6 minutes.
9. Allow the Instant Pot to automatically switch to "Keep Warm" after the timer goes off and leave it to naturally release the pressure for about 20 minutes.
10. Carefully open the lid and remove your pot de crème. Set it aside to cool for a few minutes before refrigerating for about 5 hours.
11. Serve and enjoy!

Strawberry Cobbler

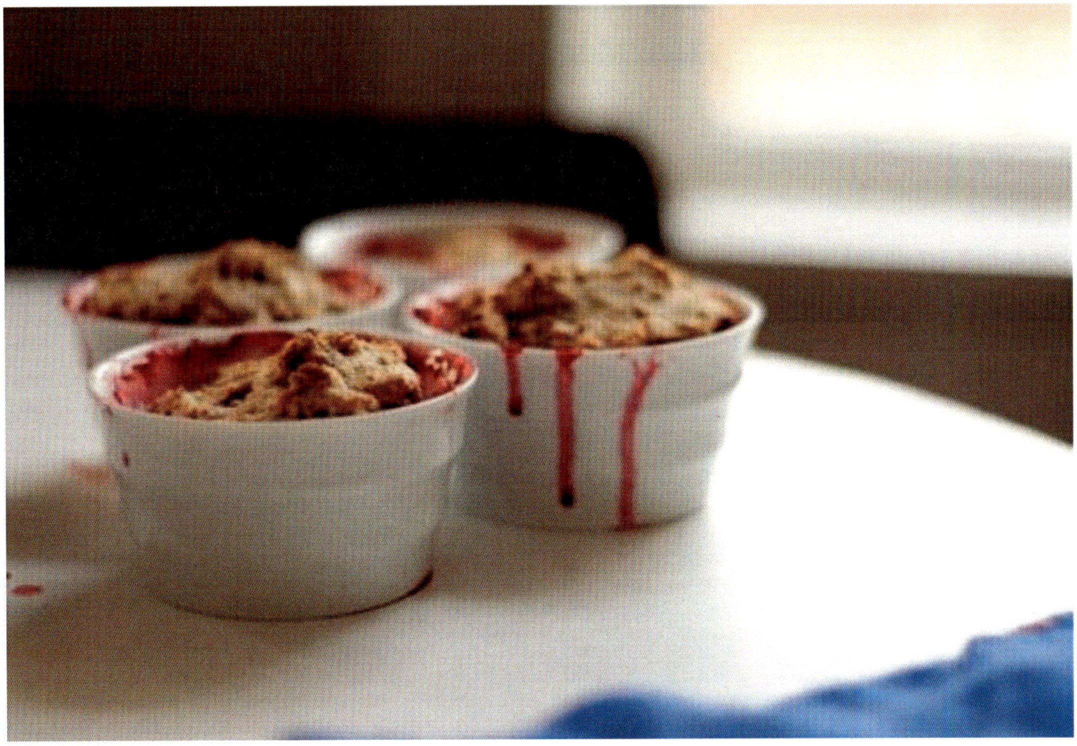

Prep Time: 5 minutes. Cook Time: 12 minutes. Total Time: 17 minutes.

Forget the traditional peach cobbler flavor and instead try out a Strawberry Cobbler. This dessert will instantly become a hit, and kids love it. With an Instant Pot, no dessert is a disappointment especially the Strawberry Cobbler.

Servings: 2

Ingredients

¾ cup strawberries, sliced
1 ¼ cups all-purpose flour
¾ cups milk
½ cup granulated sugar
1/3 cup softened butter
1½ teaspoons baking powder
1 teaspoon vanilla

Instructions

1. Add all ingredients in a large mixing bowl except the strawberries. Use a whisk to mix the ingredients. Once all the ingredients are mixed, use a spatula to fold the sliced strawberries in the batter.
2. Grease 2-3 medium sized ramekins with non-stick cooking spray and fill them the strawberry mixture.

3. Set the Instant Pot to "Manual" function and cook at "High Pressure" for 12 minutes. Once the cook time lapses, allow Natural Pressure Release for about 5 minutes.
4. Carefully open the lid remove the ramekins and set aside the Strawberry cobblers to cool
5. Serve and enjoy!

Passion Fruit Pie

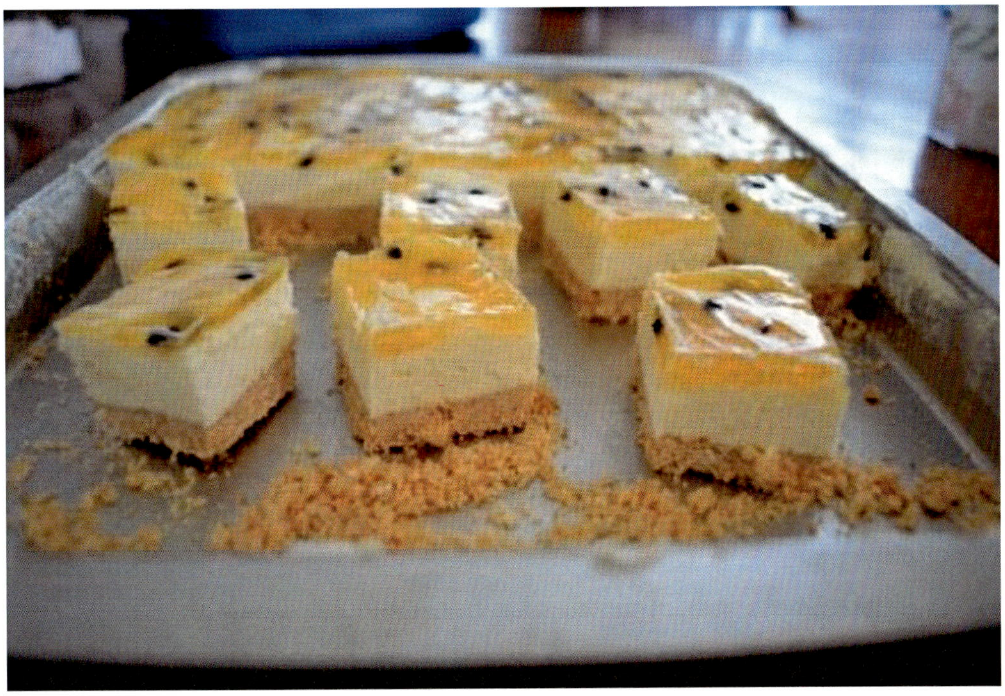

Prep Time: 6 minutes. Cook Time: 15 minutes. Total Time: 21 minutes.

Bake a delicious, exotic, creamy, citrusy, and tangy Instant Pot Passion Fruit Pie in no time. Passions fruit have a distinctive bright flavor that tastes so delicious in cakes, cookies, smoothies, mousses, and pie.

Servings: 6

Ingredients

Filling

½ cup passion fruit pulp
14 oz can condensed milk
4 large egg yolks

Crust

1 cup shortbread or butter cookies
4 tablespoons melted butter

Passion fruit coulis

¾ cup passion fruit pulp
½ cup sugar

Instructions

1. Use a non-stick cooking spray to grease a springform pan that fits in your Instant Pot.

2. Use a food processor to ground the cookies. Add the crumbled pieces of cookies and the melted butter in a mixing bowl and stir them together.
3. Make a pie crust by compacting this mixture into the sides and bottom of the pan. Place the pan in the freezer as you make the pie filling.
4. Puree the yolks, passion fruit pulp and condensed milk in a blender. Pour this creamy mixture onto the already prepared pie crust.
5. Use an aluminum foil to cover the springform pan.
6. Pour a cup of water into the Instant Pot and lower a trivet into the pot. Seal the lid.
7. Program the Instant Pot to "Manual" setting and cook at "High Pressure" for 15 minutes.
8. Allow Natural Pressure Release for 10 minutes once the Instant Pot beeps. Carefully open the lid and remove the pan. Refrigerate the pie for about 4 hours.
9. Combine sugar and passion fruit pulp in a saucepan and heat the mixture over Medium-Low heat. Stir the mixture frequently until it's reduced and thick. Refrigerate the coulis.
10. Once the passion fruit coulis has cooled, pour it on the pie, slice and serve.
11. Enjoy!

Upside-Down Apple and Ricotta Cake

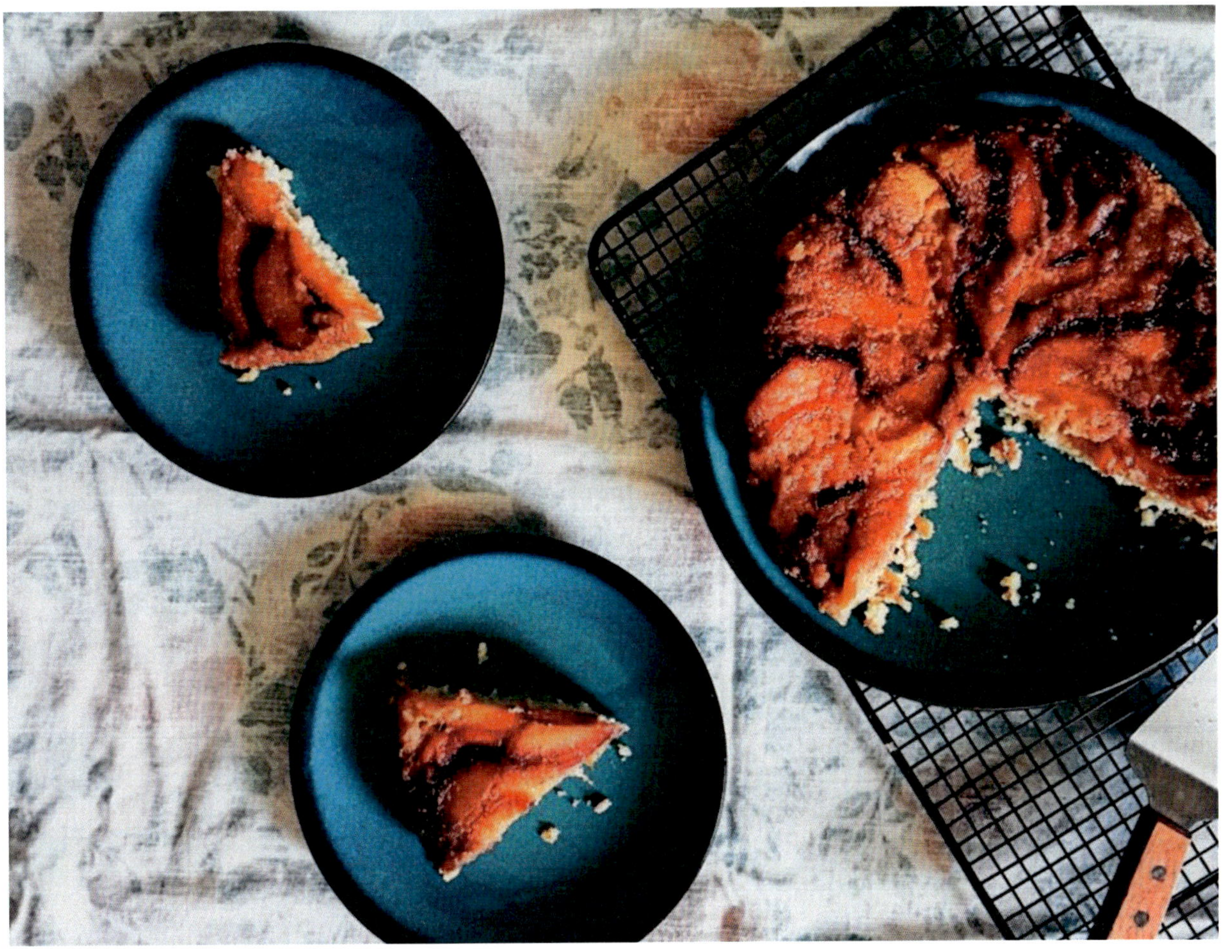

Prep Time: 10 minutes. Cook Time: 20 minutes. Total Time: 30 minutes.

This is an excellent cheese and egg-centric Apple Cake that you can easily serve over and over with tea. You can tweak the recipe by substituting apples with peaches, apricots, pears, nectarines or mandarins. Soaked raisins and crushed walnuts also make great additions to this cake.

Servings: 4

Ingredients

2 apples, 1 diced 1 sliced
1 cup ricotta cheese
1 cup all-purpose flour
2 cups water
1 egg
¼ cup raw sugar
1/3 cup sugar
2 teaspoons baking powder
1 teaspoon baking soda
3 tablespoons extra-virgin olive oil

1 tablespoon lemon juice
1 teaspoon vanilla extract (or 1 vanilla bean seeds)
1 teaspoon cinnamon

Instructions

1. Add 2 cups of water into the Instant Pot and place the steam rack.
2. Cover the diced and sliced apples with lemon juice.
3. Prepare the inner pot by placing a wax paper disc at the bottom, dusting its interior with flour and oiling.
4. Sprinkle the raw sugar in the inner pot and try to artistically arrange the sliced apple pieces.
5. Mix the egg, sugar, olive oil, ricotta and vanilla in a small mixing bowl. Sprinkle baking soda, baking powder, cinnamon and flour into the mixture using a fine mesh strainer or flour sifter.
6. Blend well the combined mixture until smooth and then stir in the diced apple pieces. Pour the mixture into the prepared inner pot and place into the Instant Pot uncovered.
7. Seal the lid and set the timer to 20 minutes at "High Pressure."
8. Allow Natural Pressure Release when the timer goes off. Unplug your Instant Pot or disengage "Keep Warm" function and unseal the lid.
9. If the cake isn't cooked through, lower it back into the Instant pot and let it cook for a few more minutes.
10. Turn the cake upside-down onto a serving plate.
11. Serve chilled or warm.
12. Enjoy!

Monkey Bread

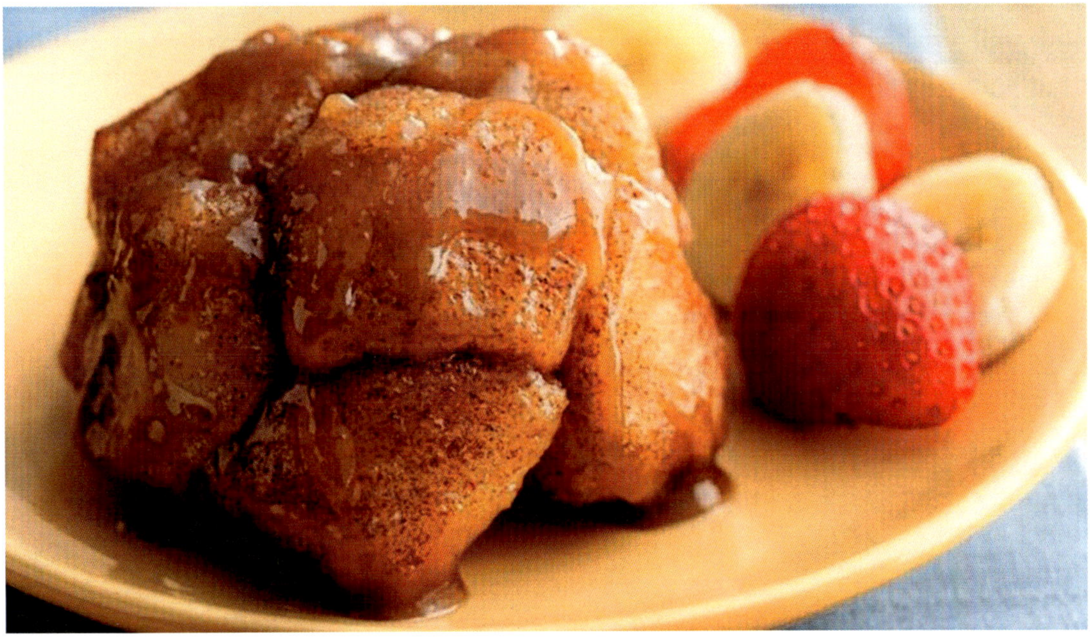

Prep Time: 3 minutes. Cook Time: 21 minutes. Total Time: 24 minutes.

Instant Pot Monkey Bread is pretty amazing. Make your Monkey Bread in the Instant Pot for a bread pudding textured outside with a warm and tasty dense inside. Unlike the baked version, Instant Pot monkey bread recipe doesn't harden and crystalize from the caramel sauce and sugar. Making it more delicious and enjoyable.

Servings: 2

Ingredients

1 can Southern buttered biscuits
1 cup water
½ cup brown sugar
½ cup sugar
½ stick butter
1½ teaspoon cinnamon

Instructions

1. Add sugar and cinnamon in a large mixing bowl and combine well
2. Break 4 biscuits into quarters and place into the sugar mixture. Thoroughly coat the biscuit pieces and place in a mini loaf pan
3. Repeat this process and place the sugar-coated biscuit pieces into the other loaf pan.
4. In a small bowl place sugar and butter and melt them in the microwave. Once melted stir to combine the mixture then evenly divide the butter and sugar mixture between the two loaf pans.

5. Pour a cup of water into the Instant Pot then place the steam rack trivet into the pot. Cover the loaf pans with a piece of foil before placing them on the trivet.
6. Seal the lid. Set the Instant Pot to "Manual" setting and cook at "High Pressure" for 21 minutes.
7. Once the timer goes off allow Natural Pressure Release for about 5 minutes, then do a Quick Pressure Release. Carefully open the lid set the monkey bread aside for a few minutes.
8. Serve and enjoy!

Caramel Popcorn

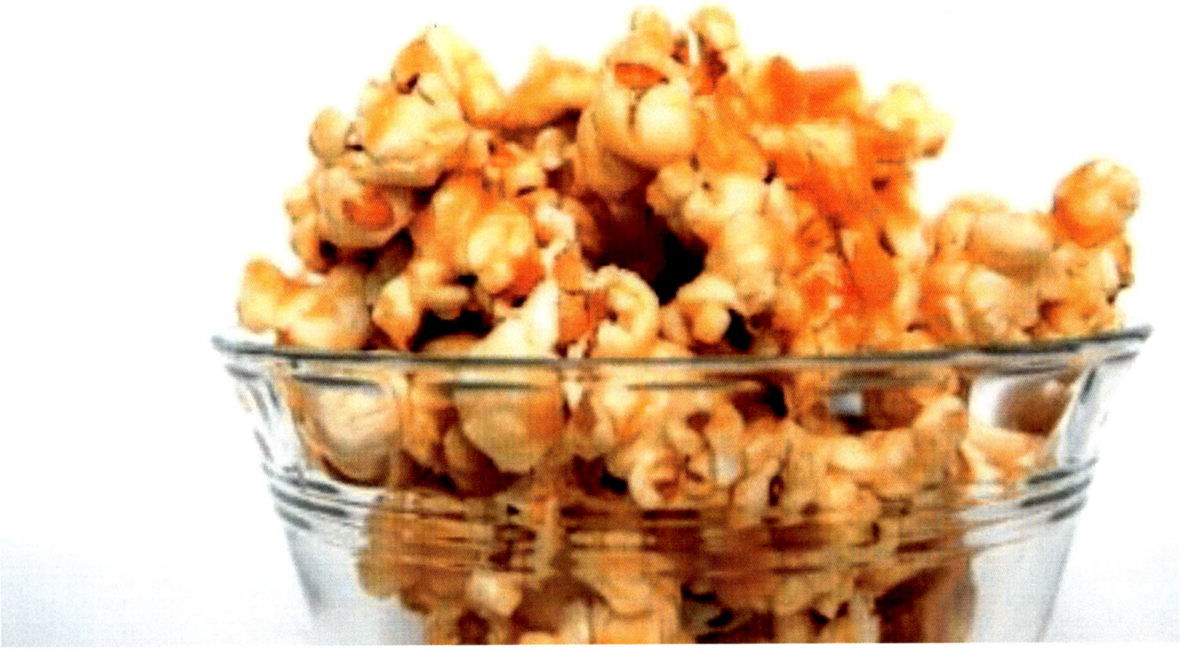

Prep Time: 1 minute. Cook Time: 5 minutes. Total Time: 6 minutes.

Flavored popcorn is always a welcomed treat. Make the ever so delicious and heavenly Caramel Popcorn for just 5 minutes, and they will be ready for a movie night. Caramel Popcorn makes a great and healthy snack so instead of chocolate make some for the kids.

Servings: 1 tub

Ingredients

½ cup corn
2 oz butter, divided
2 teaspoons coconut oil
2 teaspoons water
4 oz whole milk
2 oz white sugar

Instructions

1. Program the Instant Pot to "Sauté" function and place half the butter and coconut oil into the pot. Allow the butter and oil to heat until completely melted.
2. Pour in the corn and stir thoroughly.

3. Press "Adjust" button while the Instant Pot is still on "Sauté" mode and bring up the temperature to "Hot."
4. Close the lid once the popcorns start to pop. Wait for 2-3 additional minutes after the popping sounds stop.
5. As the corn pops, make the caramel sauce by adding 2 teaspoons of water and the sugar into a saucepan. Cook on Medium Heat until the mixture starts to turn brown. Add the remaining butter once its melted reduce the heat to Low and continue stirring. Gradually add milk to the caramel sauce until its thick enough to coat the back of your wooden spoon. Set aside to cool.
6. Remove the popcorns and carefully discard the hard bits. Transfer the popcorns into a large mixing bowl and pour in the caramel sauce, toss around the corn until they are all well-coated.
7. Refrigerate caramel popcorns for about an hour.
8. Serve and enjoy!

Coconut Yogurt

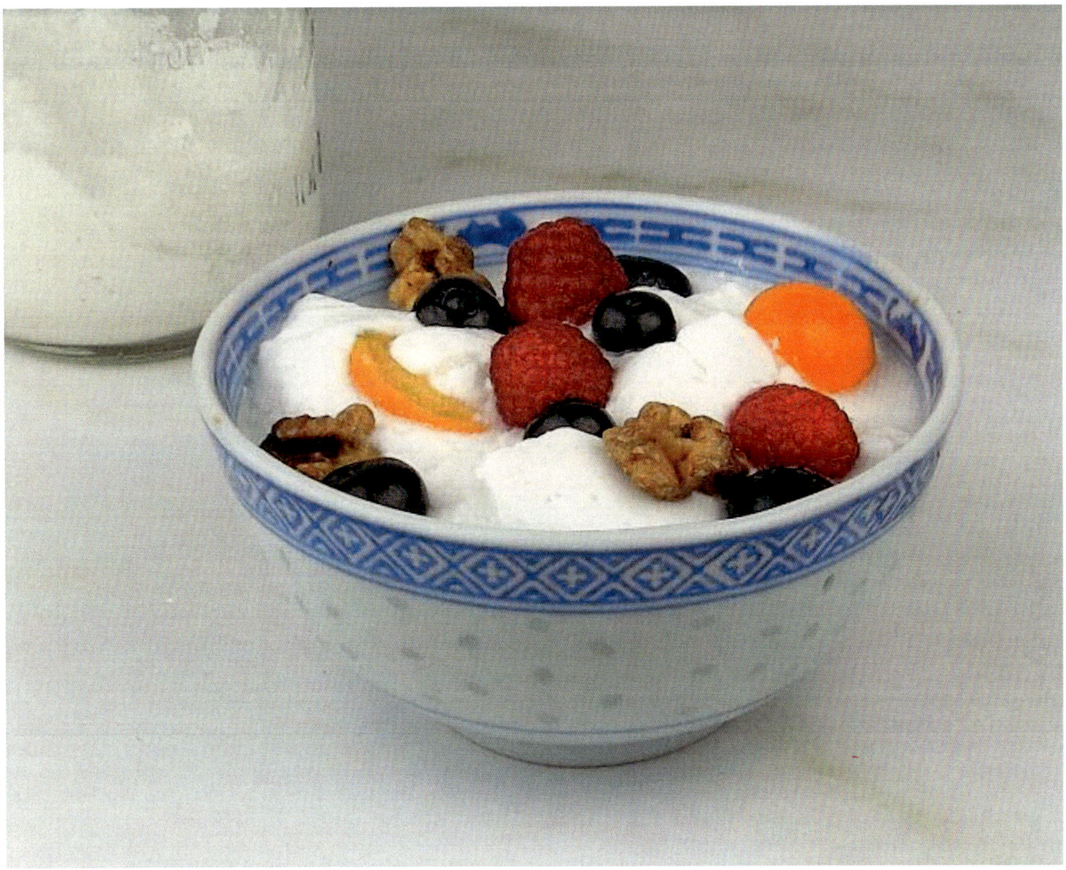

Prep Time: 5 minutes. Cook Time: 8 hours. Total Time: 8 hours 05 minutes.

If you like your yogurt Greek style, that is, plain, full fat, thick and tart then you are going to enjoy the Instant Pot Coconut Yogurt recipe. It's dairy-free and the best part you can modify the culture to make the yogurt to your desired tartness and texture.

Servings: 3-4 cups

Ingredients

1 package yogurt starter, with live cultures
2 cans coconut cream (1 liter)
1 tablespoon gelatin

Instructions

1. Pour the coconut cream into an inner pot and place it in the Instant Pot. Program the Instant Pot to "Yogurt" then "Adjust." The coconut cream will simmer to a boil.
2. Remove the inner pot once the display switches to "Yogurt." Set aside the coconut cream to cool to the desired temperature of 100F.
3. Once the liquid coconut cream cools to the right temperature, which is 100F slowly whisk in the yogurt starter. Stir until the mixture is smooth.

4. Reprogram the Instant Pot to "Yogurt" function and set the timer for 8 hours. Whisk in the gelatin.
5. Divide the yogurt equally into 3 mason jars and refrigerate for 4-6 hours.
6. Serve with your favorite toppings and enjoy!

Yogurt Crème topped with Wine Poached Figs

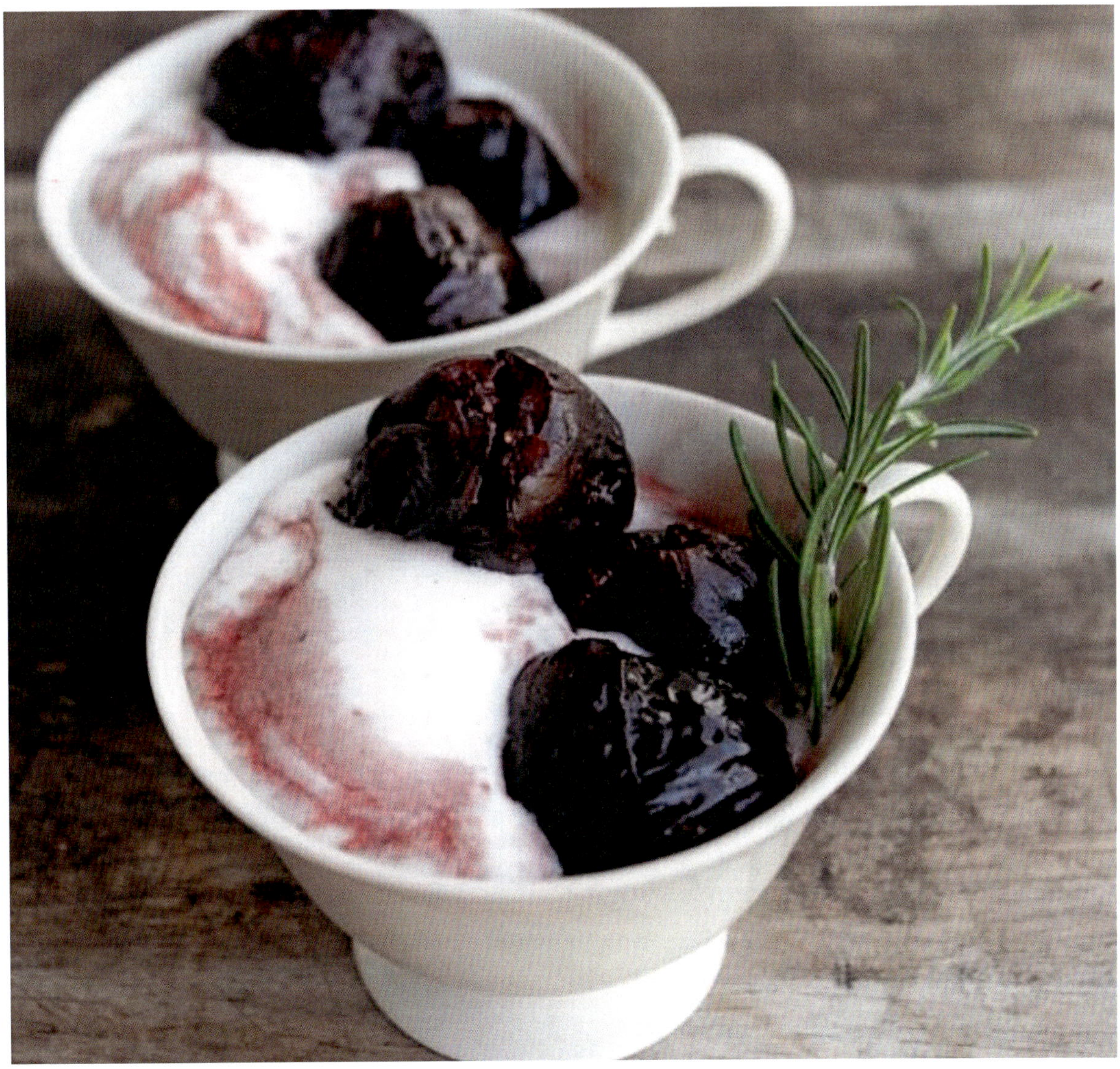

Prep Time: 5 minutes. Cook Time: 8 minutes. Total Time: 13 minutes.

The sweet and sticky figs bursting with freshness and flavor pair perfectly with crunchy pine nuts and yogurt crème. This recipe can also be served and enjoyed as a dessert

Servings: 4-6

Ingredients

2 lbs plain yogurt
1 lb figs
½ cup pine nuts
½ cup sugar or honey
1 cup red wine

Instructions

1. Use a fine-mesh strainer to sieve the plain yogurt into a bowl to make the yogurt crème. Don't press down on the yogurt just spread it out on the strainer. Then refrigerate for 4 hours.
2. As the yogurt crème cools toast the pine nuts on Medium Heat in the Instant Pot then set them aside.
3. Press on "Cancel" function then pour a cup of red wine into the Instant Pot. Place the figs in a steamer basket and place it in the Instant Pot without a steam rack.
4. Seal the lid and cook at "Low Pressure" for 3 minutes. Once the timer goes off, allow Natural Pressure Release.
5. Remove the steam basket carefully and set it aside. Add ½ cup honey or sugar into the Instant Pot and mix it with the wine to make a wine syrup. Continue stirring until the wine is reduced to half.
6. Top the yogurt crème with figs, a drizzle of wine syrup and pine nuts then serve.
7. Enjoy!

SOUPS

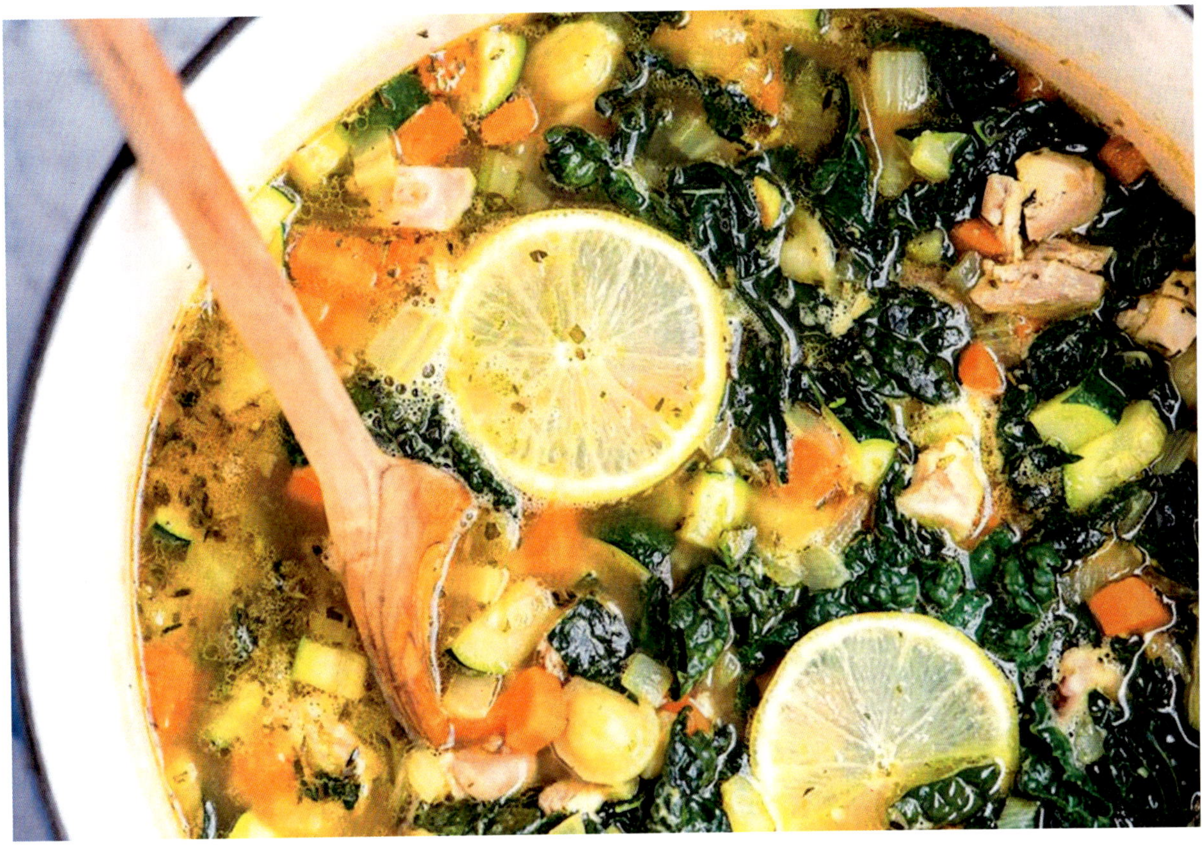

We all have those go-to soup recipes, cleaning-out-the-fridge soup recipes or our childhood favorites but is always a fun experience experimenting out of your culinary comfort zone. Instead of spending hours on end turning low-flavor, high-sodium canned varieties into soup it's time to put your Instant Pot to good use. Prepare any top-rated soup in the Instant Pot and enjoy a no-fuss comfort food. There is nothing an Instant Pot can't handle, and soups are undoubtedly one of the pot's strongest suits. Whether you enjoy the adventurous recipes, or you just want to stick with the classics, we have all your favorite and family-friendly soup recipes. All it takes to satisfy your soup craving is a bit of meal prep and a push of a button for a piping hot bowl of tasty, healthy and delicious soup.

Chicken Noodle Soup

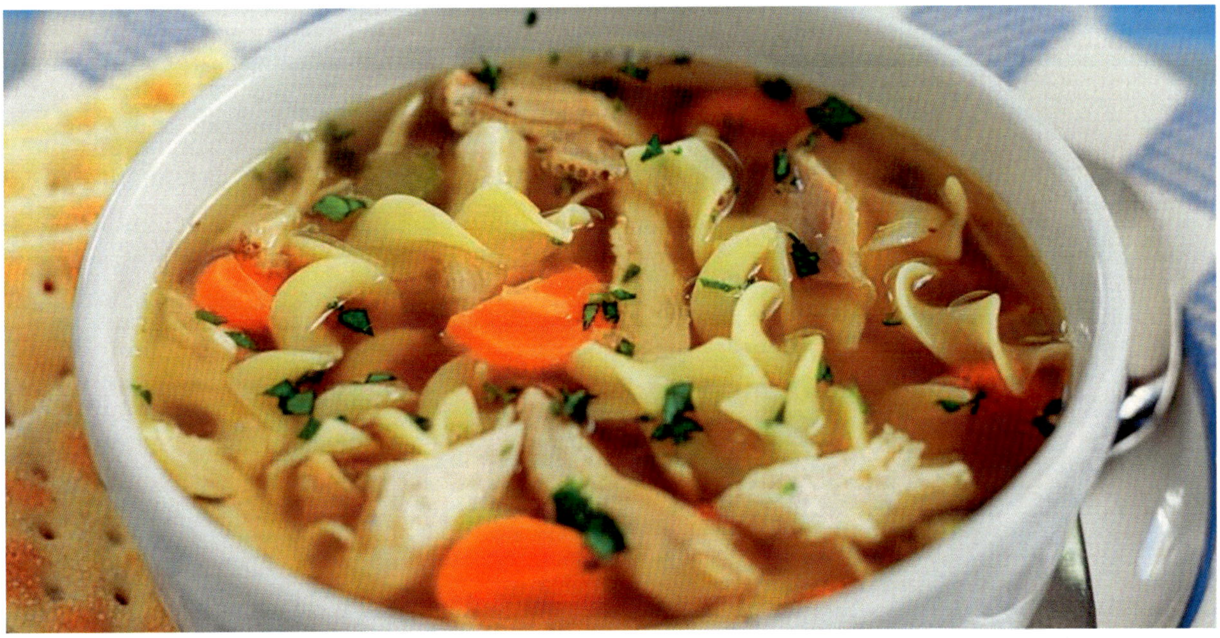

Prep Time: 10 minutes. Cook Time: 20 minutes. Total Time: 30 minutes.

The Instant Pot Chicken Noodle Soup is one of the easiest and the best soup to make. The soup is flavorful with tender chicken chunks, big hearty veggies in the rich chicken broth. Make this dish from scratch in less than an hour in the Instant Pot.

Servings: 6-8

Ingredients

5 lbs chicken, giblets removed
4 oz egg noodles, extra wide
1 tablespoon olive oil
8 cups water
1 small onion, finely chopped and diced
2 cloves garlic, finely minced
2 celery sticks, sliced into ½ inch pieces
5 carrots, peeled and sliced into ½ inch pieces
½ cup fresh flat leaf parsley, minced
2 tablespoons soy sauce
Freshly ground pepper and kosher salt, to taste

Instructions

1. Program the Instant Pot to "Sauté" function.
2. Add the olive oil to the Instant Pot. Once hot, add the onions and sauté for 2-3 minutes until they are soft and translucent.
3. Add garlic, carrot, and celery in the pot and sauté for another minute.

4. Place the whole chicken into the Instant Pot then pour in the 8 cups of water followed by soy sauce, freshly ground pepper and kosher salt.
5. Cancel the "Sauté" settings and close the lid. Ensure the Pressure Release Valve is set to "Sealing" position. Set the Instant Pot to "Manual" setting and cook at "High Pressure" for 20 minutes.
6. Allow Natural Pressure Release for about 15-20 minutes once the timer goes off. Do a Quick Pressure Release before carefully opening the lid and remove the whole chicken. Set the chicken aside to shred.
7. Program the Instant Pot back to "Sauté" function. Let the chicken broth come to a boil and stir in the egg noodles. Cook for about 5 minutes.
8. As the noodles cook, shred the chicken into desirable pieces then discard the skin and bones.
9. Stir in the chicken and fresh parsley once the noodles are cooked. If need be, add more salt and pepper to taste.
10. Serve and enjoy!

Butternut Cauliflower Soup

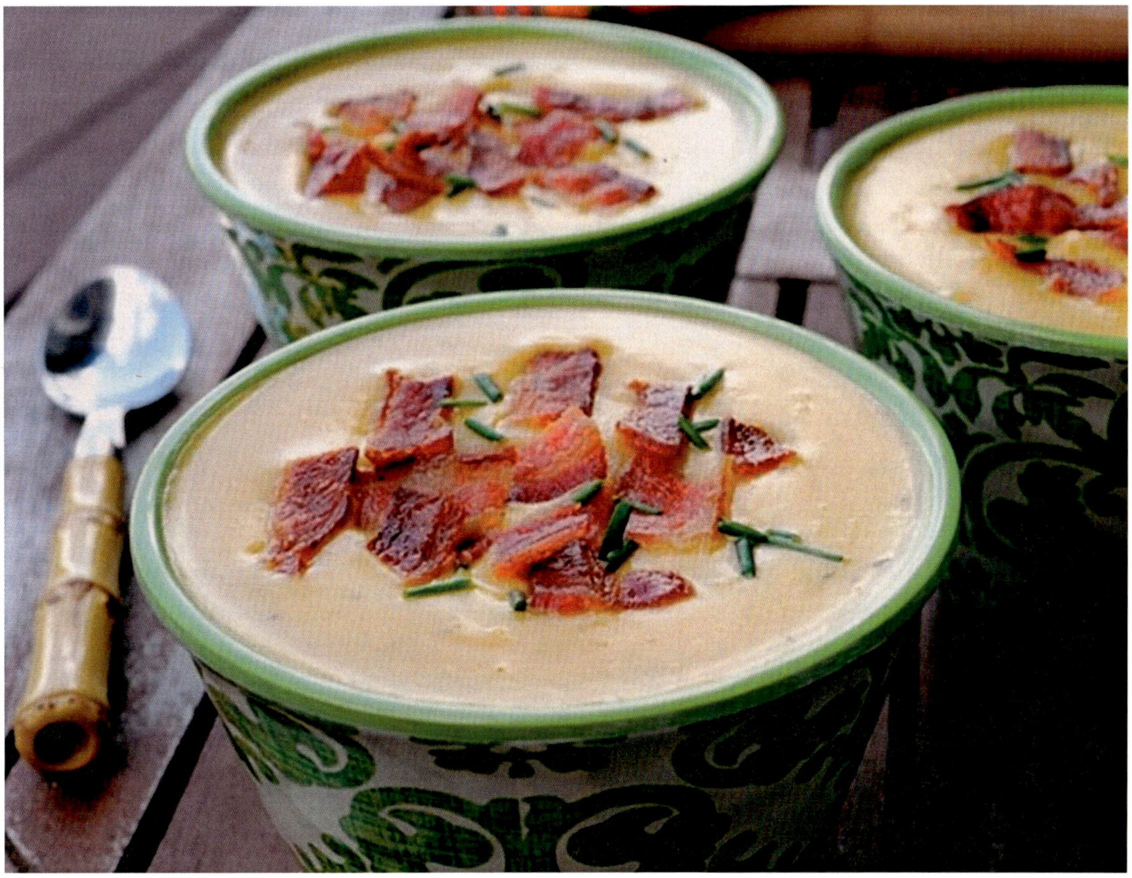

Prep Time: 15 minutes. Cook Time: 10 minutes. Total Time: 25 minutes.

While everyone is out snagging a pumpkin spice latte in homage to the fall season how about curling up indoors with a bowl of Butternut Cauliflower Soup. This heaping bowl of comforting perfection is quick and easy to make with minimum prep. Forget the ever-daunting task of peeling and chopping the hard butternut squash by using pre-chopped butternut. The tasty soup with tons of flavor will not only be a fall favorite but a go-to comfort food this and every fall.

Servings: 6

Ingredients

1 lb frozen cubed butternut squash
1 lb frozen cauliflower
2 cups chicken or vegetable broth
½ cup milk or cream
1-2 teaspoon oil
1 onion, finely diced
2-3 cloves garlic, minced
1 teaspoon paprika
½ - 1 teaspoon dried thyme
¼ teaspoon sea salt, to taste

¼ - ½ teaspoon red pepper flakes (optional)

Mix-ins and topping options

Crumbled bacon
Parmesan and/or gouda cheese
Grated cheddar cheese
Chopped green onions
Sunflower seeds
Pumpkin seeds
Hot sauce or sriracha
Pesto
Croutons
Chives, sour cream and cheddar cheese

Instructions

1. Set the Instant Pot to "Sauté" function and heat up the oil.
2. Add onions in the Instant Pot and sauté them until tender and golden then add garlic and cook for a few seconds.
3. Add butternut, cauliflower, veggie or chicken broth and the spices.
4. Close the lid and ensure the Pressure Release Valve is set to "Sealing" position. Set the Instant Pot to "Manual" function and cook at "High Pressure" and cook for 5 minutes.
5. Do a Quick Pressure Release once the timer goes off and carefully open the lid. Then stir in ½ cup of milk or cream.
6. Allow the soup to cool before blending it into a smooth mixture. Use either blender or a food processor or a blender.
7. Serve the soup and top with your choice of mix-ins and toppings.
8. Enjoy!

Spicy Carrot Soup

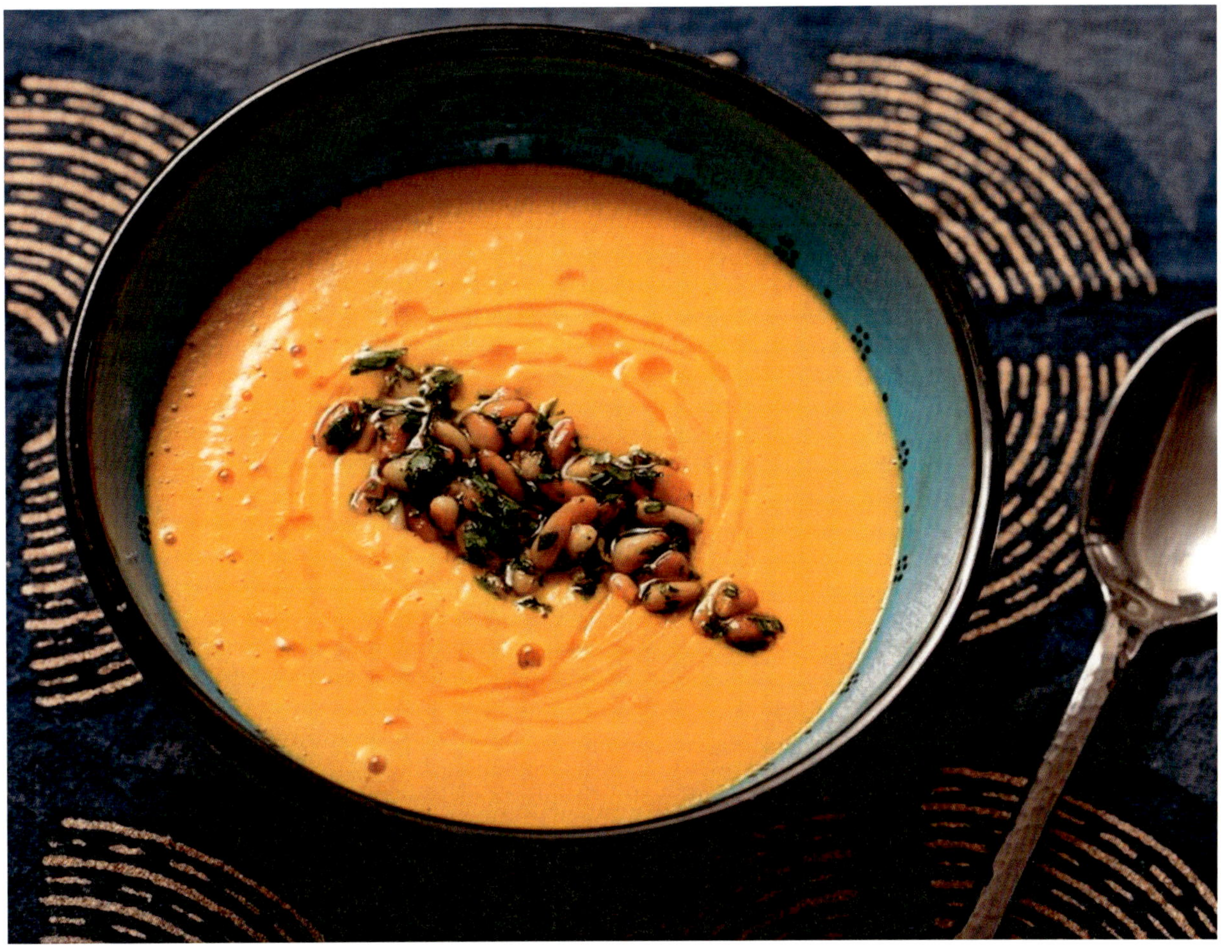

Prep Time: 15 minutes. Cook Time: 15 minutes. Total Time: 30 minutes.

The spicy carrot soup is a 7-ingredient easy curry like twist to the comfort food. The spicy Instant Pot Spicy Carrot Soup is a healthy, velvety and extremely smooth and a great addition to your favorite recipes. Spicy Carrot Soup is also freezer-friendly

Servings: 4-6

Ingredients

- 8-10 large carrots, peeled and roughly chopped
- 1½ cups chicken or veggie broth
- 14 oz can coconut milk
- 1 cup peanut butter
- 1 onion, chopped
- 3 cloves garlic, peeled
- 1 tablespoon red curry paste
- Salt to taste

Toppings

Peanuts
Cilantro

Instructions

1. Add all the ingredients into the Instant Pot.
2. Close the lid and ensure that the Pressure Release Valve is on "Sealing" position.
3. Set the Instant Pot on "Manual" setting and cook at "High Pressure" for 15 minutes.
4. Do a Quick Pressure Release once the timer goes off then carefully open the lid.
5. Set aside to cool for a few minutes then run the mixture through the blender until it's smooth and creamy.
6. Generously season the soup with salt and top with cilantro and peanuts.
7. Serve and enjoy!

Italian Wedding Soup

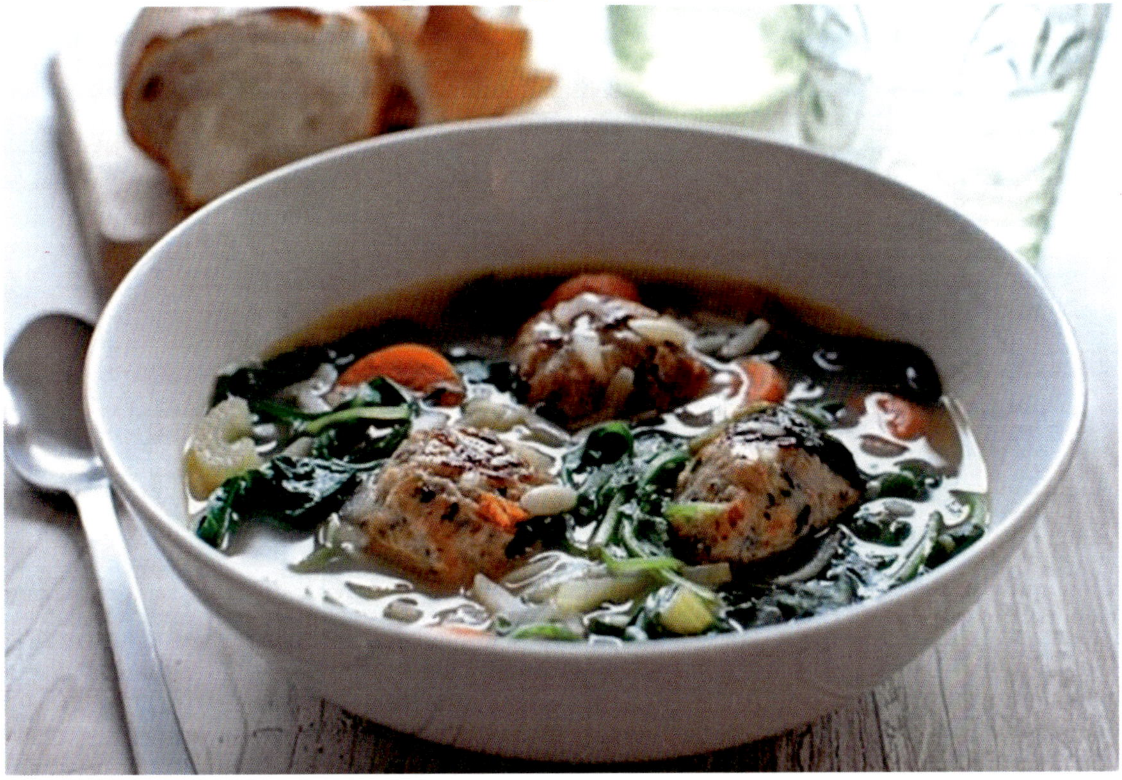

Prep Time: 10 minutes. Cook Time: 10 minutes. Total Time: 20 minutes.

If you are looking to try a healthy, low carb, gluten free, Whole30 and paleo recipe, this Instant Pot Italian wedding soup is the perfect recipe for you. The great thing about this wholesome dish is that cooking it is a breeze!

Servings: 6

Ingredients

1 lb Italian sausage
4 cups unsalted chicken stock, gluten free
2-3 cups baby spinach
2 large carrots, thinly sliced
1 large onion, finely chopped
1 clove garlic, minced
1 tablespoon olive oil
4 tablespoons parmesan cheese, grated
¼ teaspoon salt
½ teaspoon pepper

Instructions

1. Shape Italian sausage meat into small and equal sized meatballs then set them aside. A pound of Italian sausage will yield about 15 meatballs.
2. Program the Instant Pot to the "Sauté" function and adjust to the "Medium Heat" then add the olive oil.

3. Add the onions and carrots into the Instant Pot and sauté for 2-3 minutes.
4. Pour in the chicken stock then add garlic, salt, and pepper. Use a wooden spoon or a spatula to deglaze the pot and cancel the "Sauté" function.
5. Add the meatballs to the pot. Close the lid and ensure the Steam Release Vent is set to "Sealing" position. Set the Instant Pot to "Manual" mode and cook at "High Pressure" for 5 minutes.
6. Allow Natural Pressure Release for about 10 minutes once the timer goes off then do a Quick Pressure Release. Carefully open the lid.
7. Add the baby spinach leaves to the soup. Sit the lid loosely on the Instant Pot for about 2-3 minutes until the spinach is soft.
8. Serve with grated parmesan cheese.
9. Enjoy!

Instant Pot Ramen Soup

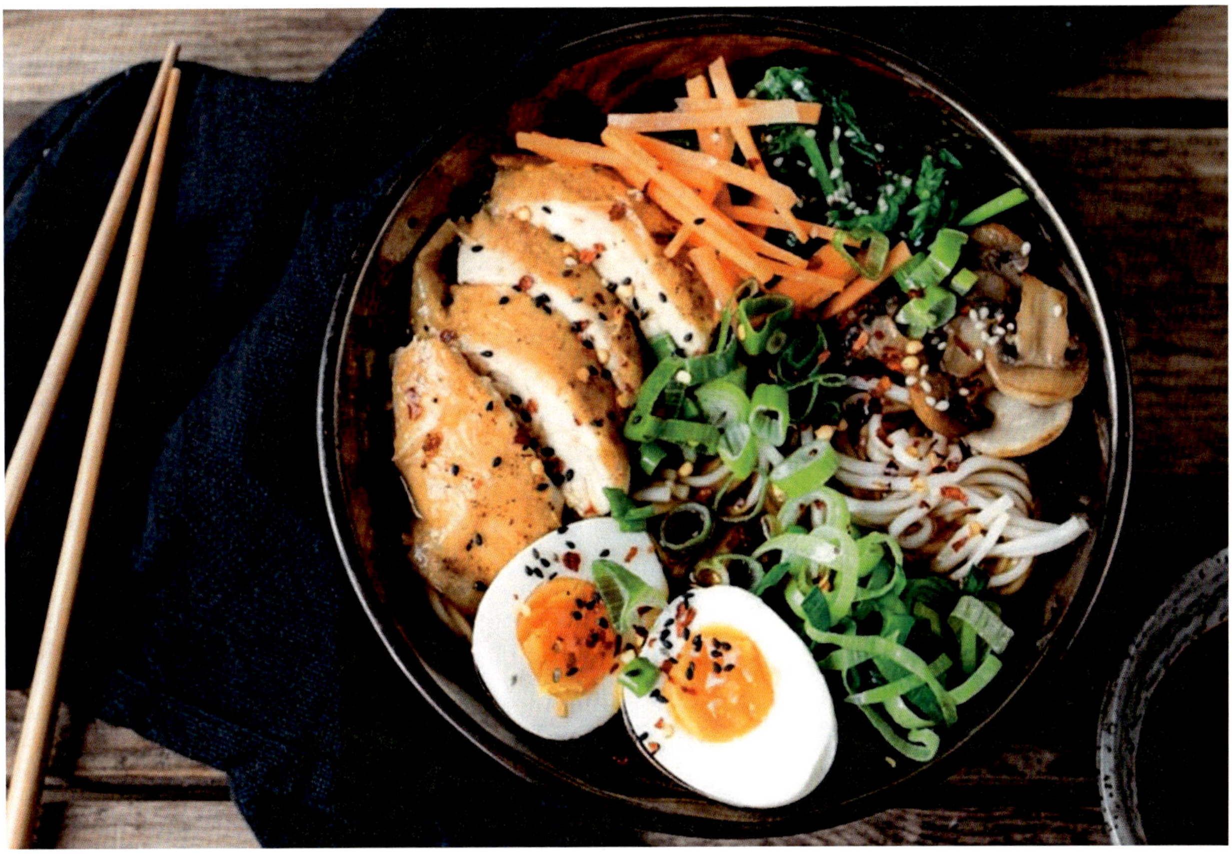

Prep Time: 10 minutes. Cook Time: 20 minutes. Total Time: 30 minutes.

The combination of mushrooms and fresh ginger creates this rich and delicious soup. Add freshly shredded carrots, baby spinach and noodles to the soup and it's already a meal. Make the soup and perfect toppings in no time in the Instant Pot.

Servings: 4.

Ingredients

1 whole (3-4lbs) chicken, giblets removed and discarded
8 oz dried ramen or udon noodles
8 oz fresh mushrooms, roughly sliced
1 cup baby spinach, thinly sliced
8 cups water
1 large carrot, peeled and grated
3 cloves garlic, minced
1 teaspoon freshly grated ginger
1 tablespoon sesame oil
2 tablespoon soy sauce
Freshly grounded pepper and kosher salt to taste.

Toppings

Soft-boiled egg
Sesame seeds (for garnish)

Instructions

Soft-boiled eggs

1. Pour 2 cups of water into the Instant Pot and place a steam basket in the pot.
2. Place 4 eggs in the steam basket. Close the lid and ensure the Steam Release Valve is set to "Sealing" position.
3. Program the Instant Pot to "Manual" function, set the timer to 3 minutes and cook at "High Pressure".
4. Do a Quick Pressure Release once the timer goes off then carefully open the lid. Remove the eggs from the Instant Pot and place them in a water bath until cooled. Set them aside.

Ramen soup

5. Program the Instant Pot to the "Sauté" function and set to "Normal Heat."
6. Heat the oil before adding in the garlic and ginger. Sauté for 1-2 minutes.
7. Add in the mushrooms then stir the pot slightly before adding the whole chicken, water, soy sauce, freshly ground pepper and kosher salt.
8. Cancel the "Sauté" function, close the lid and ensure the Steam Releasing Valve is set to "Sealing" position.
9. Set the Instant Pot to "Manual" Setting and cook at High Pressure for 20 minutes.
10. Once the timer goes off, let the Instant Pot sit in "Keep Warm" mode then turn the Pressure Release Valve to "Venting."
11. Carefully open the lid and remove the chicken and set it aside to shred.
12. Turn back the Instant Pot to "Sauté" mode. Let the chicken broth come to a boil and stir in the noodles. Let the noodles cook as per the directions on the package.
13. As the noodles cook, shred the chicken into desired pieces and discard the skin and bones.
14. Stir in the chicken meat, carrots and spinach once the noodles are cooked. If desired, add pepper and salt to taste.
15. Serve the soup with the soft-boiled eggs and garnish with the sesame seeds.
16. Serve and enjoy!

Instant Pot Minestrone

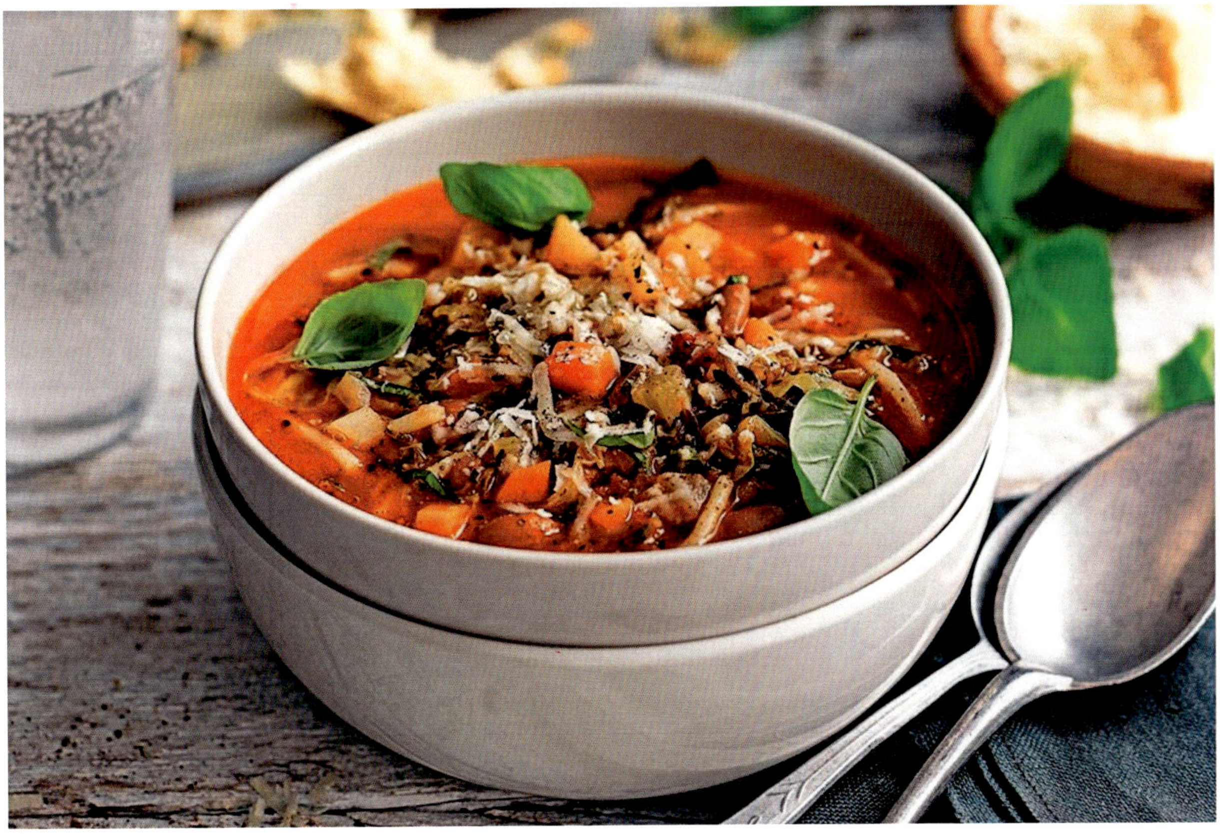

Prep Time: 20 minutes. Cook Time: 30 minutes. Total Time: 50 minutes.

Minestrone is a simple and modern-ish soup piled with lots of veggies, topped with parmesan and served with crusty bread on the side. It's a perfectly nutritious and veg-friendly soup to keep you warm during winter. This recipe can easily be made vegan.

Servings: 8

Ingredients

1 cup bulgur, uncooked
14 oz can cannellini or navy beans
24 oz marinara sauce jar
½ cup pesto
3 cups water
½ onion, finely chopped
3 cloves garlic, minced
½ head green cabbage, thinly sliced
4-5 celery stalks, chopped
4-5 carrots, peeled and chopped
3 bay leaves
2 teaspoons smoked paprika
1 teaspoon salt

Toppings

Parmesan cheese
Fresh parsley, chopped

Instructions

1. Place all the ingredients except the uncooked bulgur and the toppings in the Instant Pot. Close the lid and program the Instant Pot to the "Soup" function and set the timer for 30 minutes.
2. Do a Quick Pressure release once the timer goes off, carefully open the lid. Fish out all the bay leaves from the pot and discard them. Add in the bulgur and loosely replace the lid. To cook the bulgur, allow the pot to sit for about 20 minutes. If needed add more water.
3. Top your soup with parmesan cheese and garnish with freshly chopped parsley.
4. Enjoy!

Broccoli Cheddar Soup

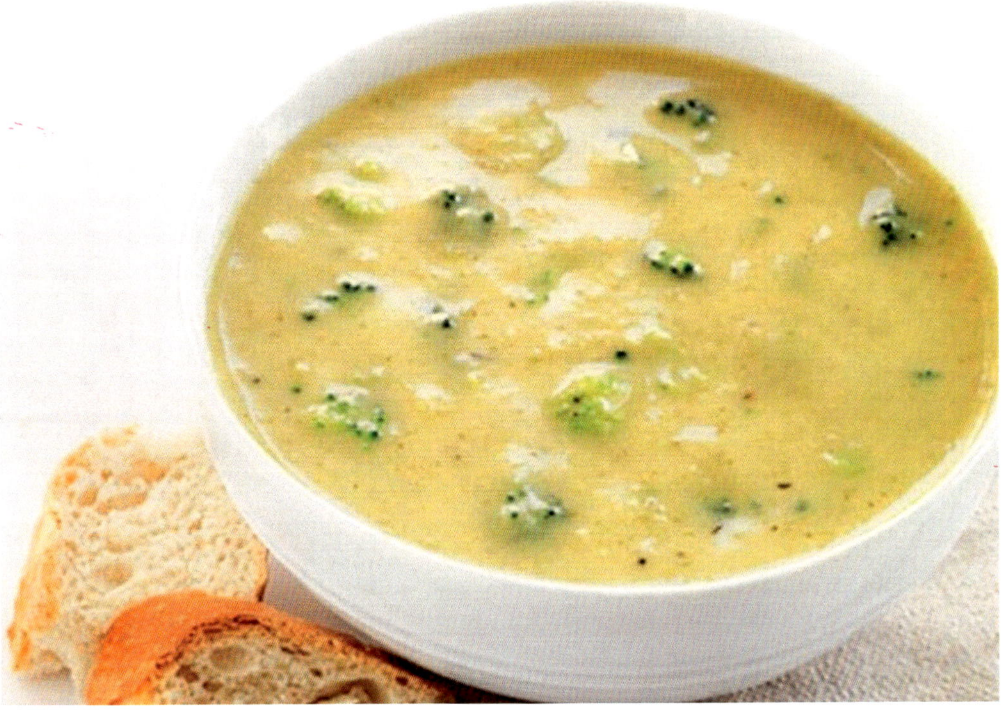

Prep Time: 5 minutes. Cook Time: 8 minutes. Total Time: 13 minutes.

Broccoli Cheddar soup is the fastest, and a more "handoff" way to turn broccoli into a nutritious and wholesome kid-friendly and family approved comfort food. Enjoy this "green awesomeness" with a loaf of bread.

Servings: 4.

Ingredients

6 cups broccoli florets
2 carrots, roughly chopped
½ onion, finely chopped
4 cups chicken bone broth
¼ cup heavy cream
1½ cups cheddar cheese, grated
1 tablespoon olive oil
1 teaspoon garlic salt

Instructions

1. Hit the "Sauté" setting on the Instant Pot and heat up the olive oil. Add the onions once the oil is hot and sauté for 2-3 minutes until translucent.
2. Cancel the "Sauté" function, then add in the broccoli, carrots and the chicken bone broth.
3. Seal the lid and program the Instant Pot to "Manual" setting and cook time of 4 minutes at "High Pressure."

4. After the timer goes off allow a Natural Pressure Release, the carefully open the lid. Pour the contents in a blender, add garlic salt and cream then blend until smooth and creamy.
5. Add the cheddar cheese and stir until melted. If desired adjust seasonings and serve.
6. Enjoy!

Instant Pot Carnitas Soup

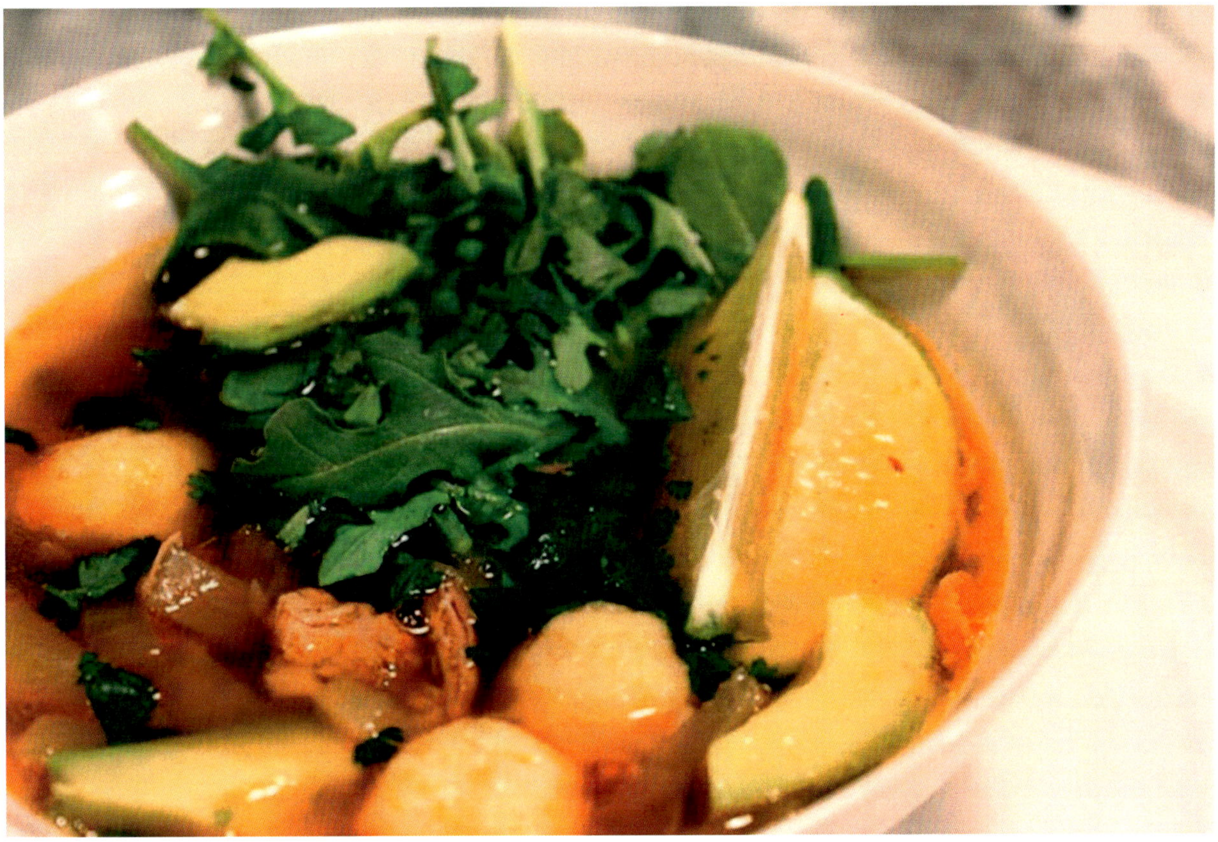

Prep Time: 10 minutes. Cook Time: 8 minutes. Total Time: 18 minutes.

Turn your leftover carnitas into a big gorgeous bowl of fresh, flavor-packed soup guaranteed to keep you warm. With only 5 required ingredients the Instant Pot Carnitas Soup is quick and easy-to-make soup recipe that you will enjoy recreating in your kitchen over and over.

Servings: 4.

Ingredients

3-4 cups carnitas
1 lb Yukon golden potatoes, diced into 1-inch pieces
16 oz (2 cups) Salsa Verde
6 cups chicken stock
2 teaspoon ground cumin

Toppings (Optional)

Pepperjack cheese, grated
Fresh arugula
Fresh cilantro, chopped
Jalapenos or serranos, sliced
Avocado, sliced

Instructions

1. Add the carnitas, potatoes, salsa verde, chicken stock and cumin in the Instant Pot. Stir to combine the ingredients and close the lid.
2. Ensure the Pressure Releasing Knob is set to "Sealing" Position. Press the "Manual" function then "High Pressure" and set the timer for 8 minutes.
3. Do a Quick Pressure Release once the timer goes off. Open the lid carefully then add seasoning if desired.
4. Serve warm with your favorite toppings.
5. Enjoy!

Instant Pot Cajun Chili

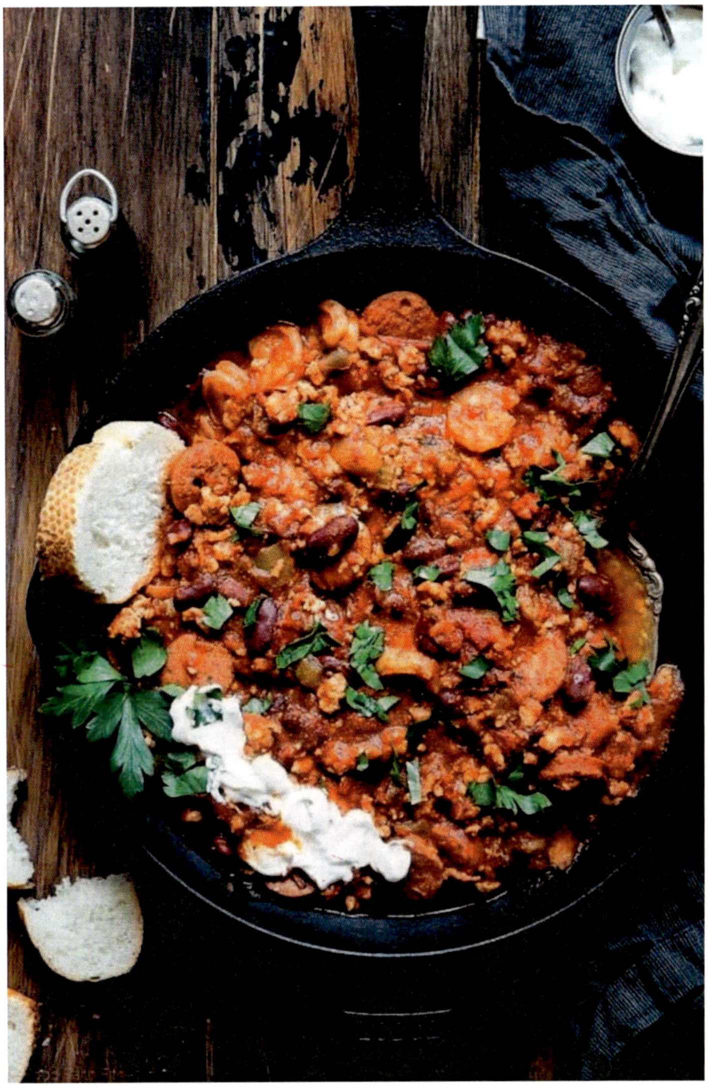

Prep Time: 15 minutes. Cook Time: 30 minutes. Total Time: 45 minutes.

With a little Cajun flair to it, the Instant Pot Cajun chili is full of addicting spicy notes of cayenne pepper and paprika, zesty punches of garlic and laced juicy bursts of ground chicken, andouille sausage and tender shrimp flavors. Enjoy the cozy warm feel with Cajun chili even when it's not warm out there anymore.

Servings: 7

Ingredients

2 links andouille sausage, sliced
1 lb ground chicken or turkey
7 oz. raw shrimp, peeled and deveined
15 oz can red kidney beans, drained and rinsed
14 oz can fire roasted tomatoes
14 oz crushed tomatoes

2 bay leaves
1 green pepper, finely diced
1½ tablespoons olive oil, divided
½ cup onion, diced
1/3 celery, diced
2 tablespoons tomato paste
1 tablespoon fresh garlic, minced
½ teaspoon sea salt
2½ tablespoons Cajun seasoning
Fresh parsley, for garnishing

Optional (for garnish)

Greek yogurt
Sour cream

Instructions

1. Program the Instant Pot to "Sauté" function, heat 1 tablespoon of the olive oil then add in onion, garlic, green pepper and celery. Cook for about 4 minutes until they begin to soften.
2. Add the ½ tablespoon of olive oil and put the chicken in the Instant Pot. Cook the chicken for about 2-3 minutes until it's no longer pink. Drain out the chicken juices and discard the liquid.
3. Place in the sausage and add in the Cajun seasoning. Stir and cook the sausage for about 5 minutes, until brown.
4. Add the beans ingredients, tomato ingredients and the bay leaves and stir until all the contents are well mixed.
5. Cover the lid and ensure the Pressure Release Valve is set to "Sealing" position. Press the "Manual" setting and cook at "High Pressure" for 10 minutes.
6. Allow Natural Pressure Release once the timer goes off and open the lid carefully.
7. Turn the Instant Pot to "Sauté" function and add in the shrimp. Stir occasionally until opaque and cooked, about 5-7 minutes. The chili will have reduced and thickened.
8. Serve and garnish.
9. Enjoy!

Tomato Basil Soup

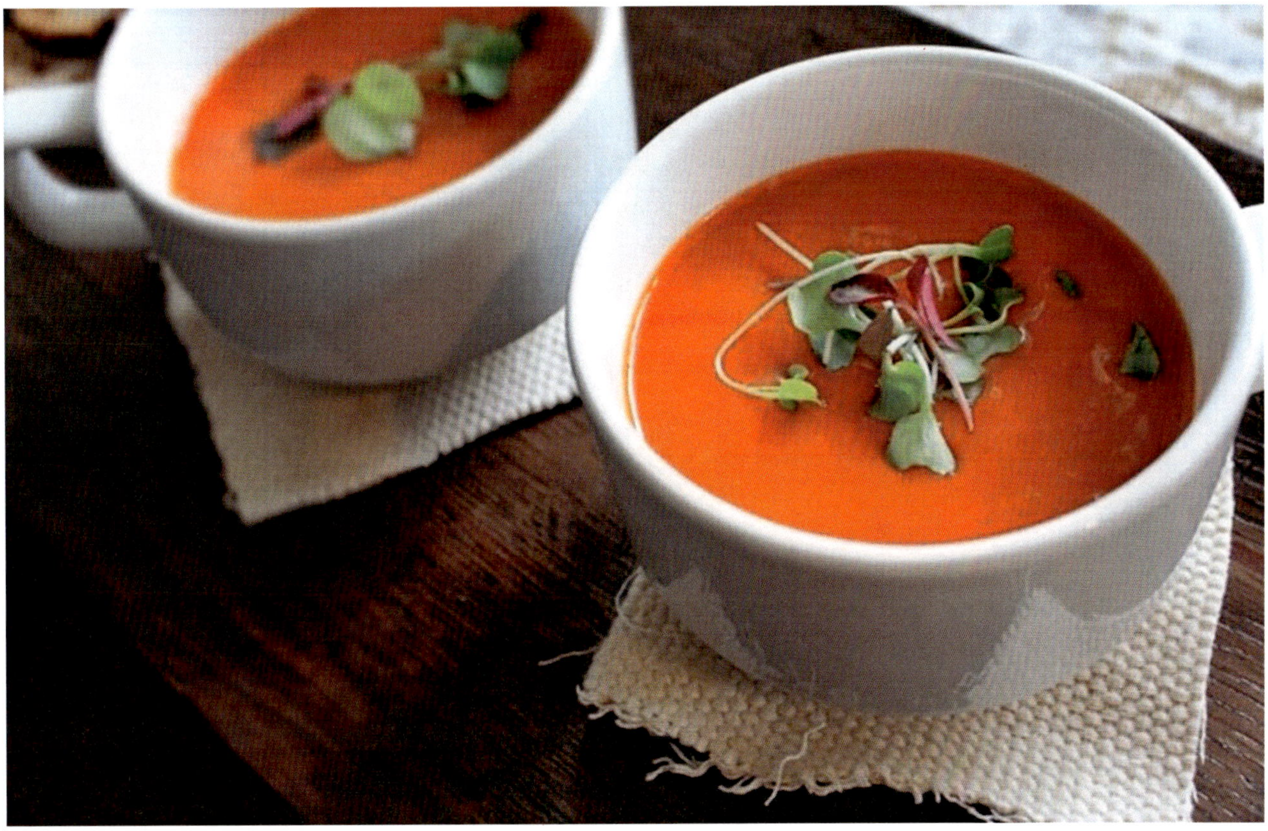

Prep Time: 5 minutes. Cook Time: 10 minutes. Total Time: 15 minutes.

If you are looking to make healthier and low-calorie meal options, the tomato basil soup is a perfect choice. With just a couple of low-calorie ingredients, you can make this flavorful soup in less than 30 minutes.

Servings: 4.

Ingredients

3 (15oz) cans diced tomatoes
1 small can tomato paste
2 cups chicken stock
¼ cup sugar
1 small onion, finely diced
1 tablespoon olive oil
1 tablespoon balsamic vinegar
1 tablespoon basil
2 teaspoons parsley
1 teaspoon garlic salt

Instructions

1. Press the "Sauté" function and heat the olive oil.

2. Add onion and tomato paste in the Instant Pot. Stir to combine the ingredients for a few minutes until the onions turn translucent and soft.
3. Cancel the "Sauté" function and add the chicken stock and the diced tomatoes.
4. Add in parsley, basil and garlic salt. Close the lid and ensure the Pressure Releasing Vent is set to "Sealing" position.
5. Program the Instant Pot to "Soup" setting and cook for 10 minutes.
6. Once the timer goes off, allow Natural Pressure Release for about 10 minutes before carefully opening the lid.
7. Stir in the sugar and balsamic vinegar.
8. Puree the contents in a blender.
9. Serve with parmesan cheese and enjoy!

Baked Potato Soup

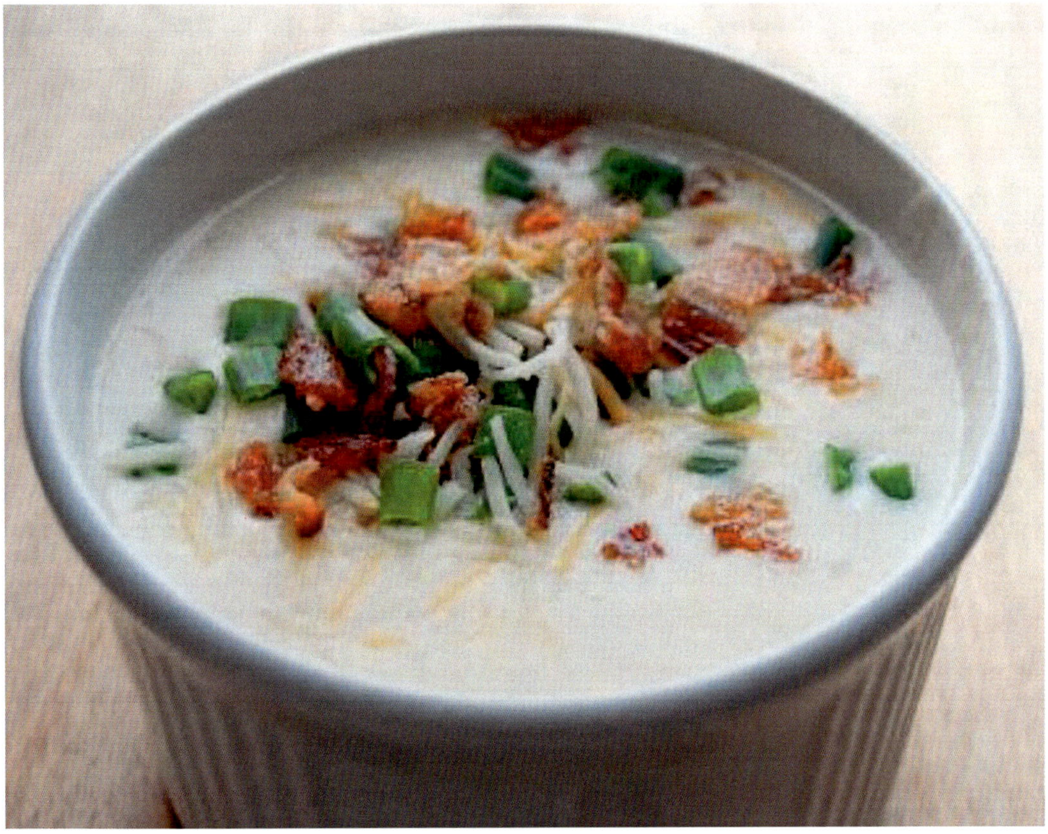

Prep Time: 15 minutes. Cook Time: 10 minutes. Total Time: 25 minutes.

With an Instant Pot, you can easily get a great homemade meal by dumping a few ingredients. The Baked Potato Soup Recipe is one of those great meals. The warm creamy and cheesy Baked Potato Soup is about to become a new hit in your kitchen. Enjoy the soup with a sandwich or some crackers.

Servings: 8

Ingredients

- 5 lbs potatoes, peeled and cubed
- 1-2 cups milk
- 2 cups cheddar cheese, shredded
- 1/3 cup softened cream cheese
- 1/3 cup sour cream
- 6 cups chicken broth
- ½ cup bacon bits, heated
- 1 large shallot, minced
- 4 tablespoons butter
- 1/8 teaspoon pepper
- ¼ teaspoon salt
- 1 green onion, finely chopped for garnish

Instructions

1. Add the potatoes, minced shallots and chicken broth. The chicken broth should cover the potatoes.
2. Seal the lid. Program the Instant Pot to "Soup" setting and cook for 10 minutes. Do a Quick Pressure Release and carefully open the lid once the timer goes off.
3. Use a large fork or a potato masher to mash the cooked potatoes. Add cheddar cheese, sour cream, cream cheese, butter, pepper and salt. Pout this mixture into a blender and puree until smooth.
4. Add the milk and stir until the soup thickens to your desired consistency.
5. Serve and top with bacon bits.
6. Enjoy!

Italian Farmhouse Veggie Soup

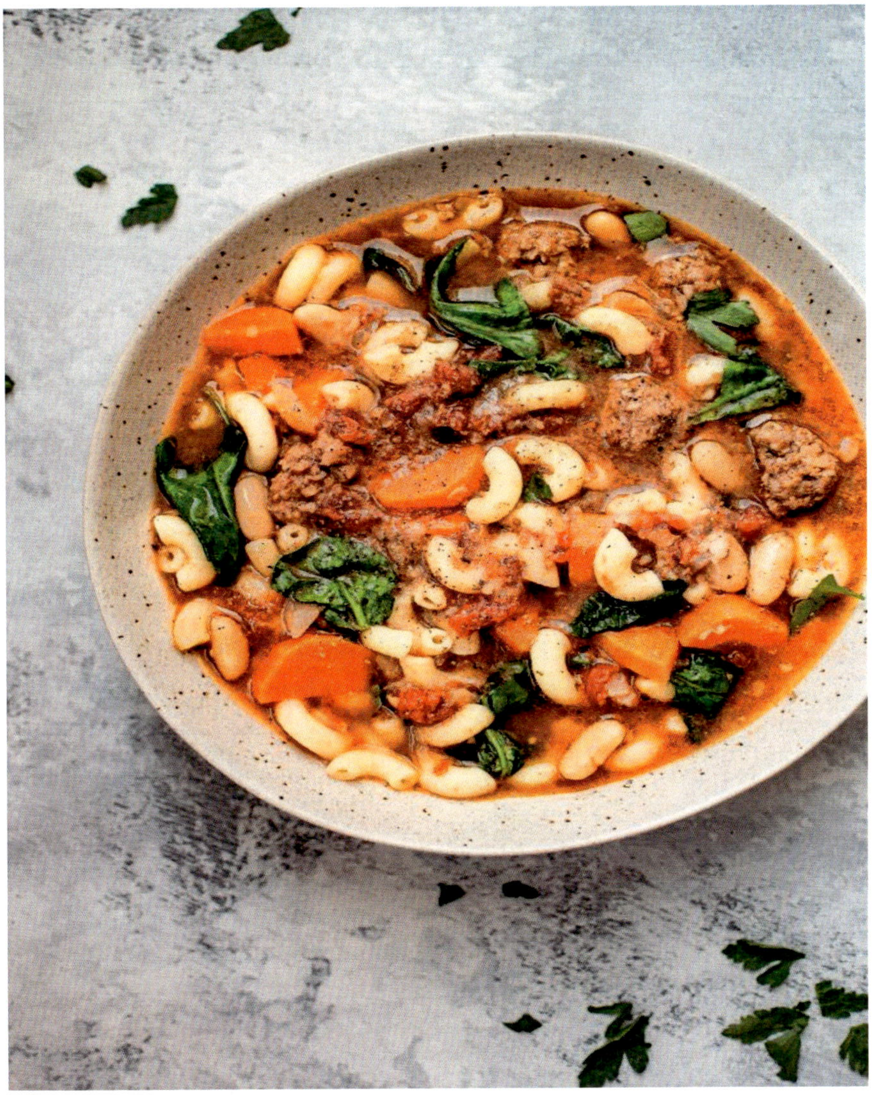

Prep Time: 10 minutes. Cook Time: 15 minutes. Total Time: 25 minutes.

For a nutritious and hearty easy-to-make soup try out the Italian Farmhouse Veggie Soup. The Italian-inspired bowl of soup is a tasty vegan and lighter meal option bursting with flavorful goodness.

Servings: 4

Ingredients

6 large button mushrooms, sliced
Handful forest mushrooms or dried porcini mushrooms
1 cup tomato passata or chopped tomatoes
3-4 oz kale leaves or cavolo nero
2 medium carrots, peeled and sliced
1 small zucchini, diced
2 celery sticks, diced

1 bay leaf
1 brown onion, diced
4 cloves garlic, diced
½ long red chili, sliced
4 cups chicken or vegetable stock
1 tablespoon olive oil
¼ teaspoon salt
Chopped parsley and lemon zest for garnish

Instructions

1. Program the Instant Pot to "Sauté" function and allow the pot to heat up.
2. Add oil, celery, onions, carrots, and salt into the pot, stir and let them cook for 1-2 minutes.
3. Add chili, garlic and all the mushrooms then stir then cook for an additional 2 minutes.
4. Finally add the stock, bay leaves, kale, tomatoes, and zucchini and give the pot another stir.
5. Press the "Cancel" function then seal the lid. Program the Instant pot to "Manual" setting and set a timer for 10 minutes.
6. Allow Natural Pressure Release once the timer goes off then do a Quick Release to ensure all the steam.
7. Serve and garnish with the lemon zest and chopped parsley.
8. Enjoy!

Bean and Beef Chili

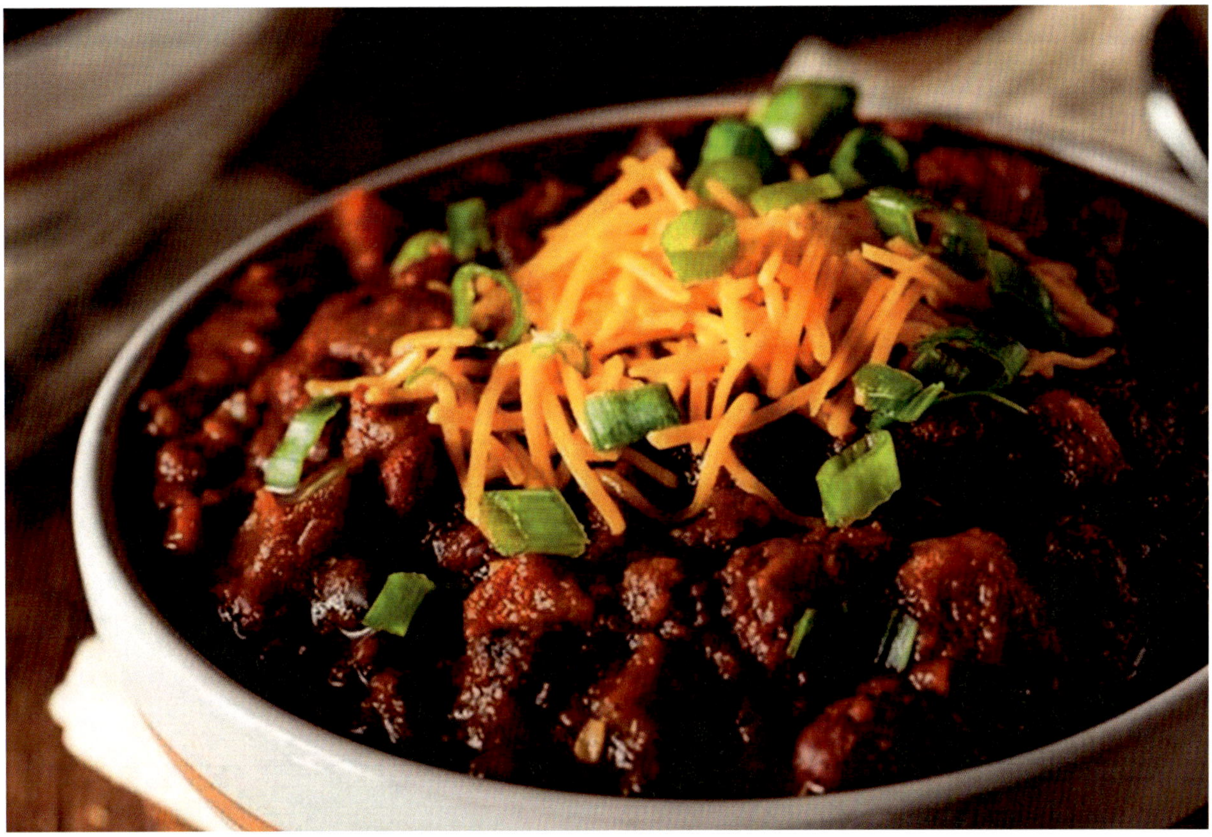

Prep Time: 10 minutes. Cook Time: 35 minutes. Total Time: 45 minutes.

This simplified Instant Pot Chili dish is not only an easy enough option for a weeknight dinner but a great addition to dinner parties. It takes only 45 minutes to make the perfectly cooked beans with juicy ground beef bursting with flavors and brighten by grated cheddar cheese, diced jalapeno and green onions will give you a satisfying fill of hearty comfort food. This under-an-hour recipe is freezer-friendly so you can make it ahead and serve later.

Servings: 4-6

Ingredients

1-1½ pound ground beef
2 cans (19 oz) red kidney beans, drained and rinsed
1 can (28 oz) crushed tomatoes
4 garlic cloves, minced
1 medium onion, finely diced
1 tablespoon olive oil
1-2 tablespoons chili powder (depending on your preference)
1 tablespoon cumin seed, grated
1 teaspoon oregano, dried

Optional

1 tablespoon apple cider vinegar
Kosher salt, brown sugar and black pepper to taste

Chicken stock mixture

1 cup unsalted chicken stock
3 tablespoons tomato paste
2 tablespoons fish sauce
1 tablespoon light soy sauce
1 teaspoon unsweetened cocoa powder

Garnish (Optional)

Cheddar cheese
Lime, sour cream
Green onions
Jalapeno pepper, seeded and diced

Instructions

1. Press the "Sauté" button and adjust to "Medium Heat" and wait until the indicator displays "Hot."
2. Generously season the ground beef with black pepper and salt. Add the olive oil and ensure that the oil covers the bottom of the pot before placing in the ground beef.
3. Leave the ground beef in the Instant Pot for about 5 minutes before removing the ground beef juice. Reserve the beef juice in a small mixing bowl.
4. Continue stirring the ground beef and allow it to brown and slightly crisp for about 5-7 minutes. Taste and adjust the seasoning with more ground black pepper and kosher salt.
5. Add the minced garlic, diced onions, dried Oregon, chili powder and ground cumin seeds in the Instant Pot. Sauté for 5 minutes and stir frequently.
6. While the ground beef is browning, mix the unsalted chicken stock, tomato paste, light soy sauce, fish sauce and unsweetened cocoa powder in measuring cup to make the chicken stock mixture.
7. Pour some of the chicken stock mixture into the pot and deglaze the bottom of the pot with a wooden spoon. Mix all the bits with the chicken stock mixture.
8. Add the reserved beef juice, the remaining chicken stock mixture, the crushed tomatoes and the drained kidney beans. Don't mix the combination.
9. Seal the lid and set the Instant Pot to "Manual" function, cook at "High Pressure" for 10 minutes.
10. Once the timer goes off, allow "Natural Release" and open the lid carefully.
11. If the chili gets is runny give it a stir and cook for a few more minutes. When its ready taste and season with kosher salt, brown sugar and black pepper. Add apple cider vinegar at this point if desired.

12. Garnish with chili and the optional ingredients and serve over your favorite side dish.
13. Enjoy!

BEVERAGES

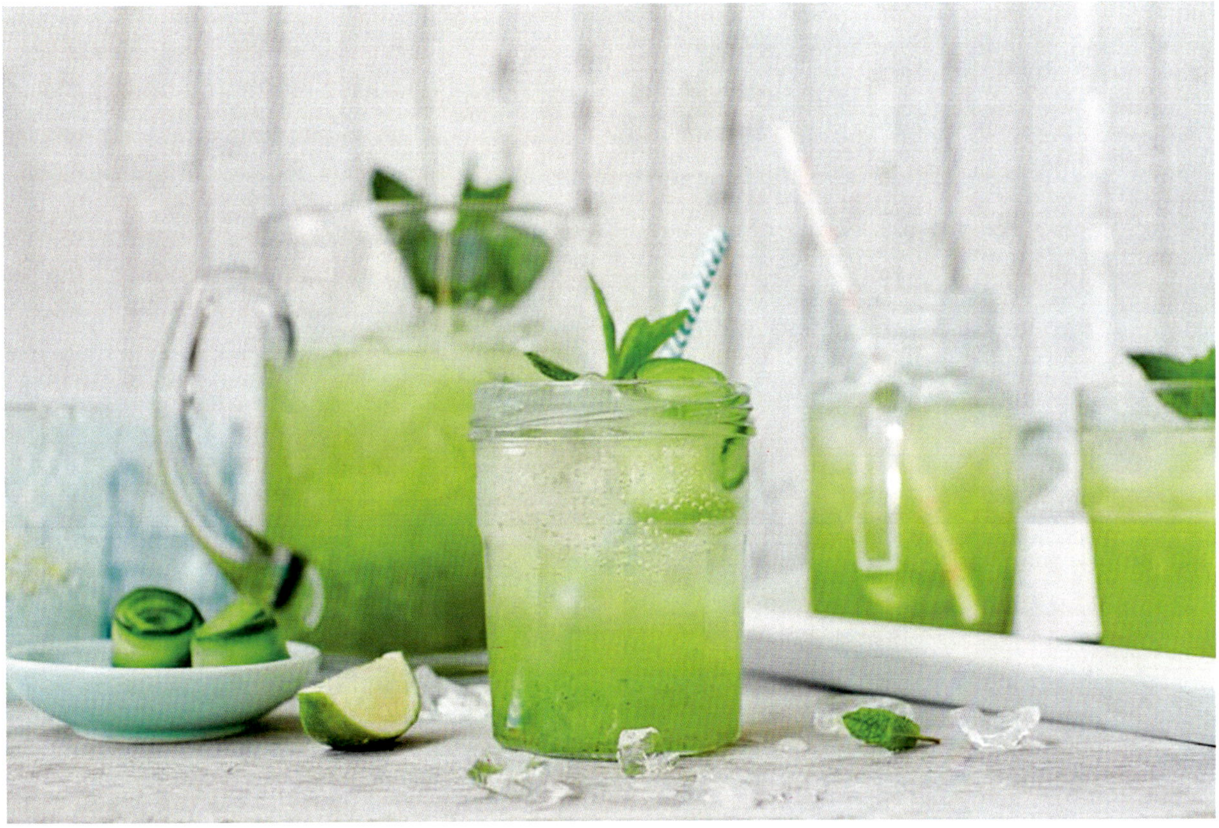

No meal is ever really complete and filling without the perfect drink. If you've had the Instant Pot, then you've probably used it to make iced tea by now. You, however, can make hot coffee drinks, mocktails, cocktails, fruity drinks and other hot or cold drinks for all occasions, ages, and celebrations in your Instant Pot. Shake things up with Instant Pot beverage recipe inspirations and make fruity favorites, refreshing classic blends and seasonal tipples. Keep your family and friends hydrated by exploring these delicious and healthy thirst-quenching recipes. They are fun, quick and easy to make. The great thing about using the Instant Pot is that you get to control the type of milk or sweetener to use as per your dietary preferences and tastes.

Cranberry Juice

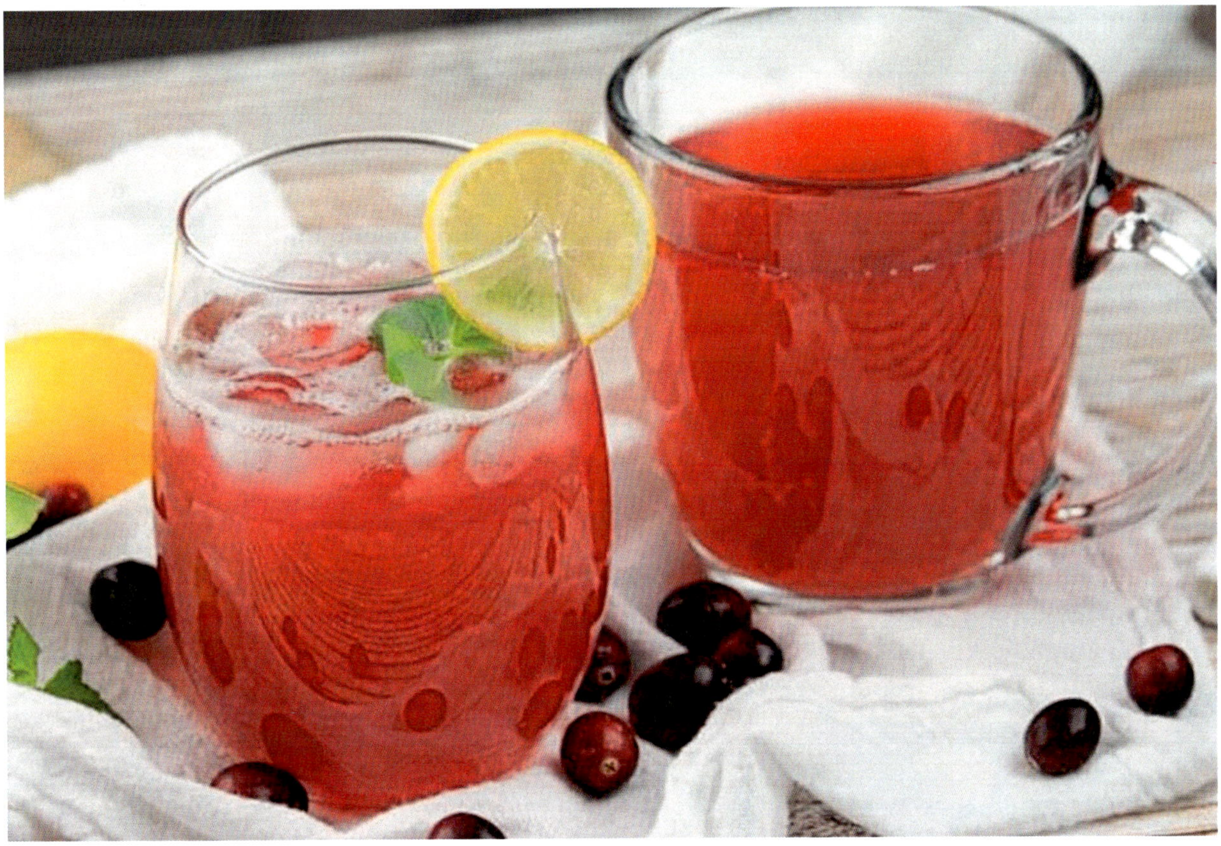

Prep Time: 5 minutes. Cook Time: 8 minutes. Total Time: 13 minutes.

Whether you enjoy a hot or an iced beverage, the slightly tart, honey-sweetened with hints of cinnamon, cranberry juice is a festive and colorful addition to your meal. The juice is freezer friendly, so make it and refrigerate for later.

Servings: 1 gallon.

Ingredients

4 cups fresh cranberries
½ - 1 cup raw honey
1 fresh lemon, juiced
1-gallon water, divided
1 cinnamon stick

Instructions

1. Pour ½ gallon of water and add the cranberries in the inner pot of your Instant Pot. Close the lid. Push the Pressure Release Knob to "Sealing" Position.
2. Program the Instant Pot to "Manual" setting and set to cook at "High pressure" and cook for 8 minutes.
3. Allow Natural Pressure Release once the timer goes off. Open the lid and carefully remove the inner pot. Set the inner pot aside to cool.

4. Once cooled strain the combination into a jar removing the cranberry pulp and the cinnamon stick.
5. Add the remaining water to the jar and set aside to continue cooling. Once cooled stir in the raw honey and freshly squeezed lemon juice.
6. Serve iced as a juice or warm as a cider.
7. Enjoy!

Peppermint Vanilla Latte

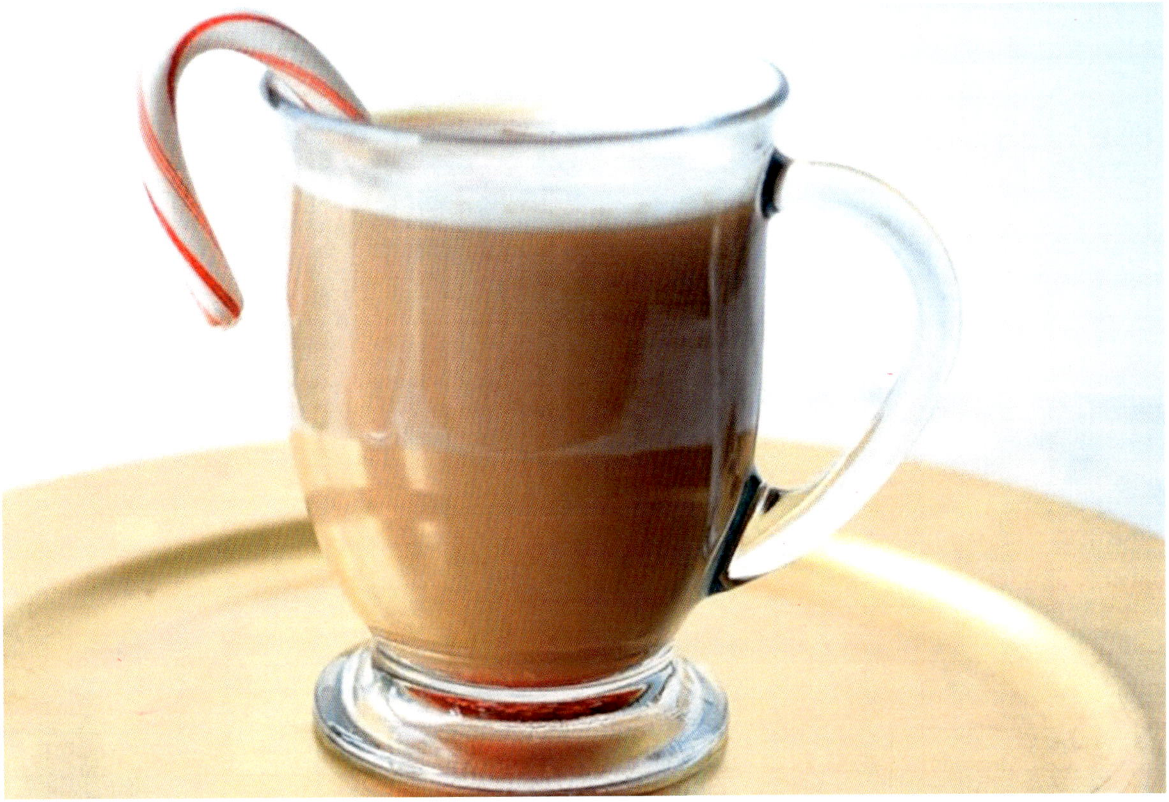

Prep Time: 5 minutes. Cook Time: 5 minutes. Total Time: 10 minutes.

This is the best drink to show off how great and versatile the Instant Pot is and leave your family and friends green with envy. The Instant Pot Peppermint Vanilla Latte recipe can also be a guideline for your coffee recipes. The Peppermint Vanilla Latte is sweet, the Instant Pot enhances and elevates its flavors making it even better.

Servings: 6-8

Ingredients

2 cups coffee or espresso shots
4 cups milk
2-3 drops peppermint essential oils
1 teaspoon vanilla
¼ cup sugar (or use any sweetener of choice)

Instructions

1. Place all the ingredients in the Instant Pot.
2. Seal the lid. Program the Instant Pot to "Manual" setting and cook at "High Pressure" for 5 minutes.
3. Once the timer goes off, allow Natural Pressure Release it will take about 10 minutes. Carefully open the lid.
4. Serve hot and enjoy!

Instant Pot Horchata

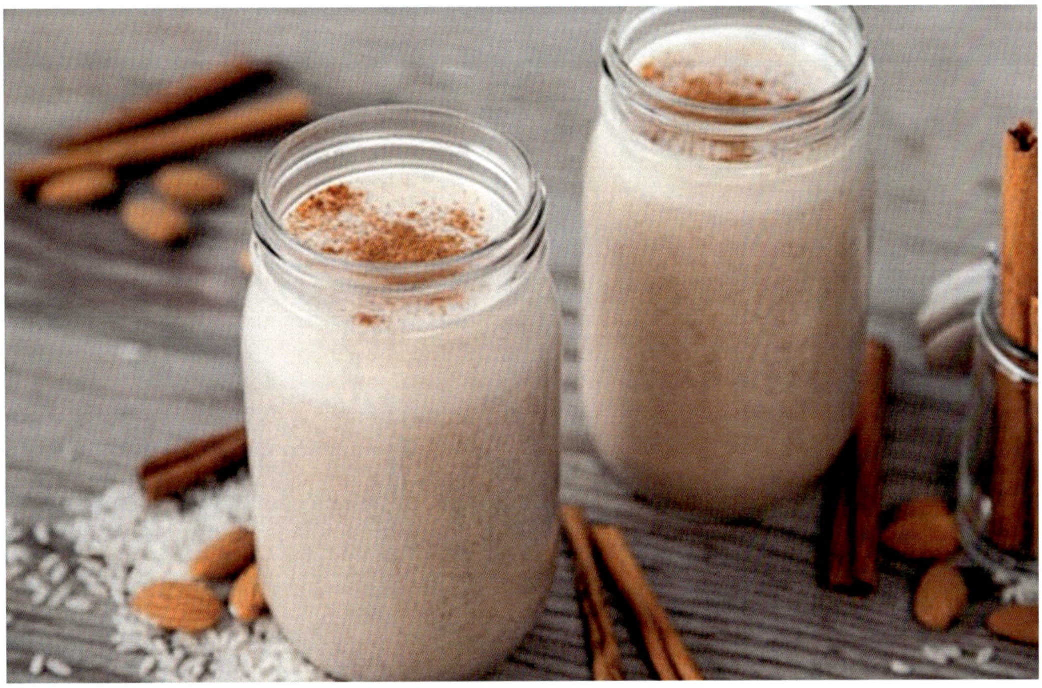

Prep Time: 5 minutes. Cook Time: 4 minutes. Total Time: 9 minutes.

Restaurant Horchata mixes are delicious and fabulous but too sugary. Infuse all the right flavors in the Instant Pot and make the perfect Horchata in the comfort of your kitchen.

Servings: 8.

Ingredients

- 32 oz unsweetened rice milk
- 1 stick cinnamon
- 6 tablespoons sugar or sweetener

Instructions

1. Pour the unsweetened rice milk into the Instant Pot then add sugar/sweetener and small chunks of the cinnamon stick.
2. Press the "Manual" setting and cook at "High Pressure" for 4 minutes.
3. Allow Natural Pressure Release once the timer goes off then do a Quick Pressure Release. Carefully open the lid.
4. Serve hot or chilled over ice and enjoy!

Mulled Wine

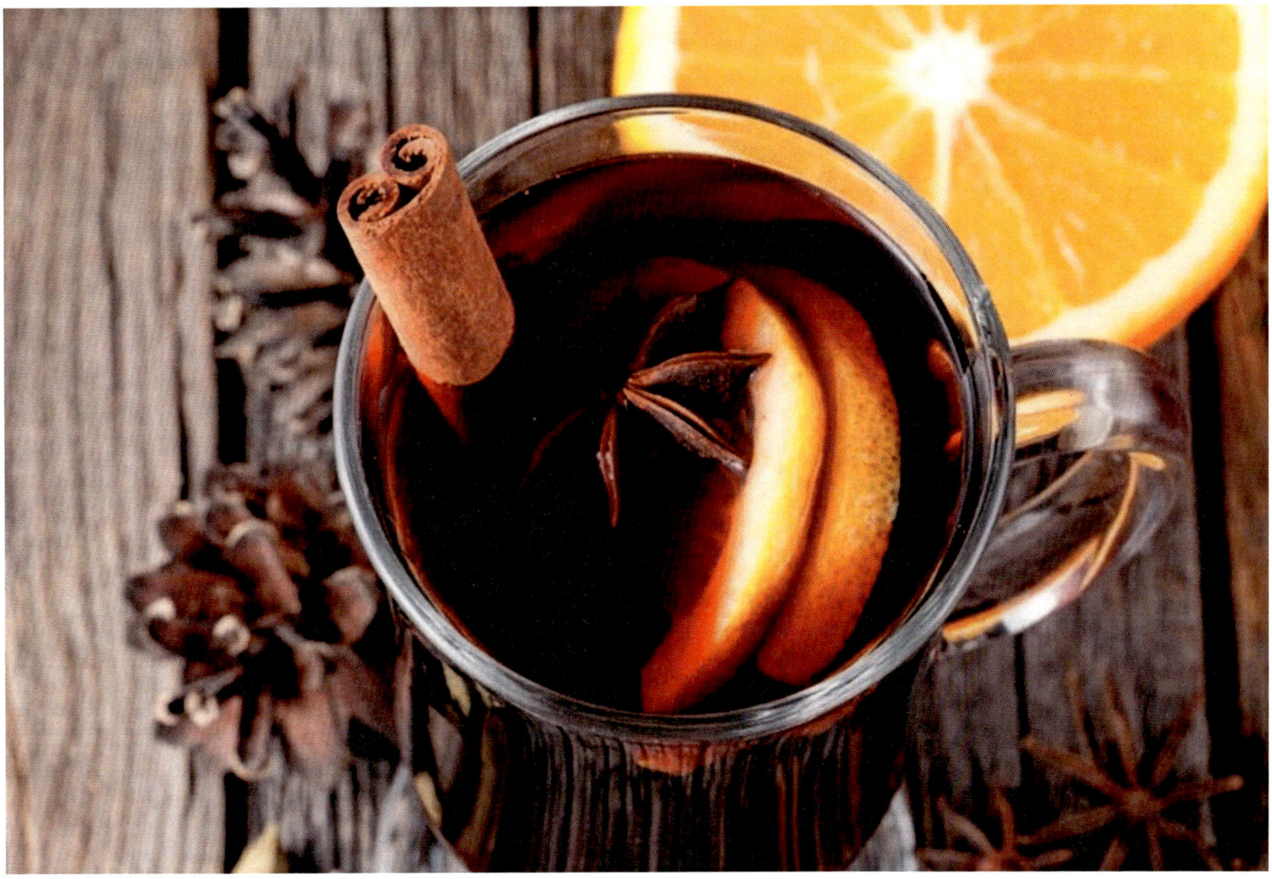

Prep Time: 15 minutes. Cook Time: 1 minutes. Total Time: 16 minutes.

One minute under pressure in the Instant Pot is all it takes to make this warm winter drink. Warm up and keep your guest entertained with this fruit and spice infused wine. Mulled wine is great for cozy get-togethers and festive parties.

Servings: 12

Ingredients

6 cups dry red wine (like Merlot, Sangiovese or chianti)
¾ - 1 cup white sugar
1 apple, thinly sliced
1 orange, sliced and cut into wedges
3 cinnamon sticks
6 juniper berries
3 Star anise
12 cloves, whole
1 teaspoon nutmeg

Instructions

1. Add all the ingredients except the orange wedges in the Instant Pot. Close the lid and ensure the Pressure Releasing Valve is set to "Sealing" position.
2. Set the Instant Pot to "Manual" setting and cook at "High Pressure" for 1 minute.
3. Do a Quick Pressure Release once the timer goes off (never allow Natural Pressure Release because it will make the mulled wine bitter and un-drinkable).
4. Carefully open the lid and stir to mix the contents in the Instant Pot.
5. Leave the Instant Pot on "Keep Warm" mode and keep enjoying the spicy mulled wine during the party.
6. Serve in a glass or mug with a speared orange wedge.
7. Enjoy!

Hibiscus Tea

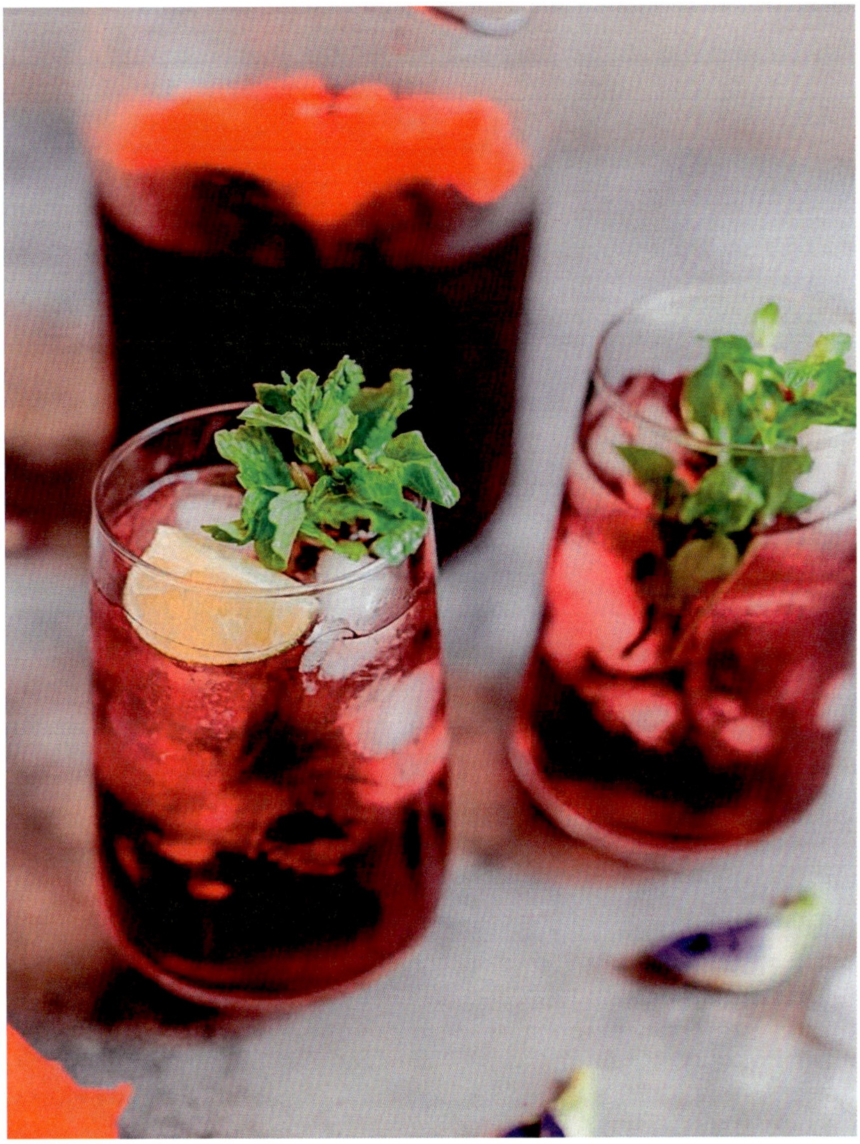

Prep Time: 10 minutes. Cook Time: 4 minutes. Total Time: 14 minutes.

Dried hibiscus leaves make a lovely, refreshing and smooth tasting deep red summer drink. The best thing about making Hibiscus Tea is that straining is a breeze because the petals easily sink to the bottom when cooked.

Servings: 8

Ingredients

1 cup hibiscus flowers, dried
8 cups water
1 cup sugar or any sweetener of choice

Optional

1 stick cinnamon

½ teaspoons minced ginger
Lime juice to taste

Instructions

1. Add all the ingredients except the lime juice in the inner pot and seal the lid.
2. Program the Instant Pot to "Manual" setting and cook at "High Pressure" for 4 minutes.
3. Allow Natural Pressure Release for about 10 minutes once the timer goes off. Do a Quick Pressure Release and carefully open the lid and remove the inner pot and set aside.
4. Once cooled, decant the liquid into a glass pitcher. For a little acidity add lime juice.
5. Serve over ice and enjoy.

Caramel Apple Cider

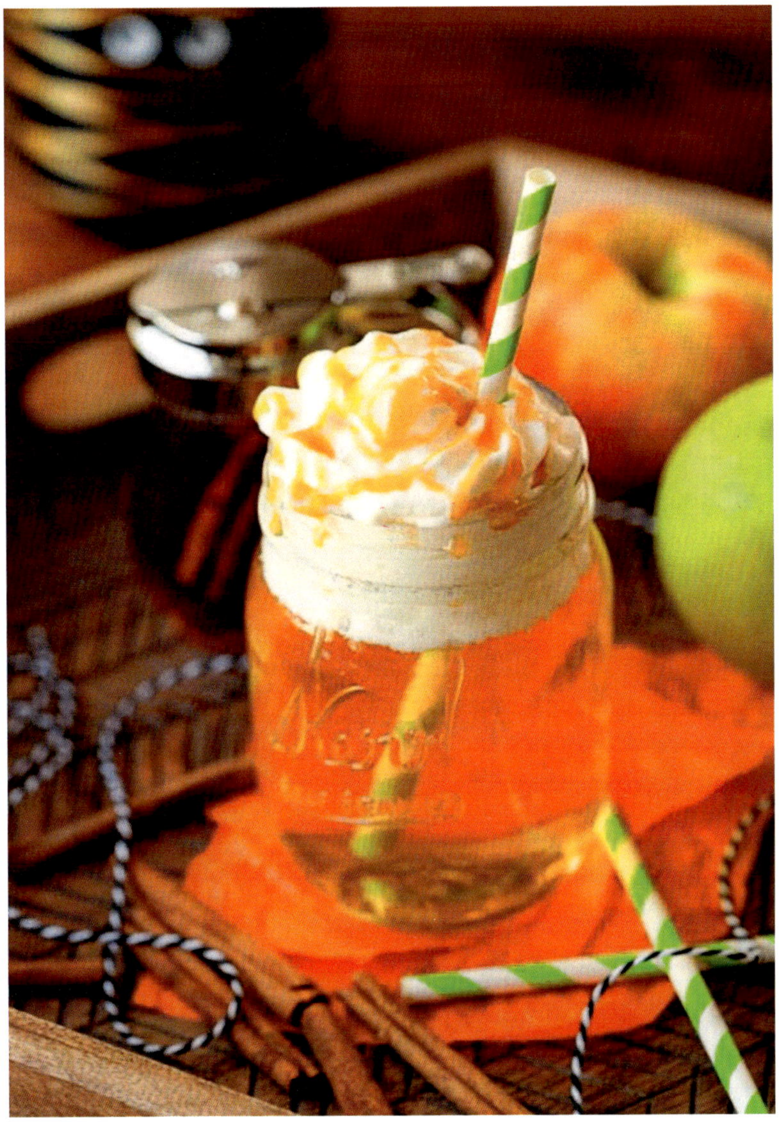

Prep Time: 15 minutes. Cook Time: 15 minutes. Total Time: 30 minutes.

Create a lighter version of everyone's favorite, the Starbuck's Caramel Apple Cider. There is no need to pile up on sugar because the apple fruit is already a sweet fruit. So no need to go overboard on the sugar.

Servings: 6

Ingredients

3 Honeycrisp apples, chopped
3 Gala apples, chopped
6-8 cups water (to completely cover the apples)
3 ground cloves
3 cinnamon sticks
3 tablespoons stevia

Toppings

Sugar-free caramel
Whipping cream
Ground cinnamon

Instructions

1. Place all the ingredients in the Instant Pot. Close the lid and ensure the Pressure Releasing Valve is set to "Sealing."
2. Set the Instant Pot to "Manual" setting and cook at "High Pressure" for 10 minutes.
3. When the timer for 10 minutes goes off, do a Quick Pressure Release and carefully open the lid.
4. Use a hand blender to puree the mixture. Ensure the blender is fully submerged and be careful not to burn yourself with the hot splashes.
5. Close the lid and continue cooking at "High Pressure" on "Manual" setting for 5 minutes.
6. Then do a Quick Pressure Release. Carefully open the lid and use a strainer to strain the mixture.
7. Serve the apple cider topped with whipped cream, cinnamon, and caramel.
8. Enjoy!

8 Infused Water recipes

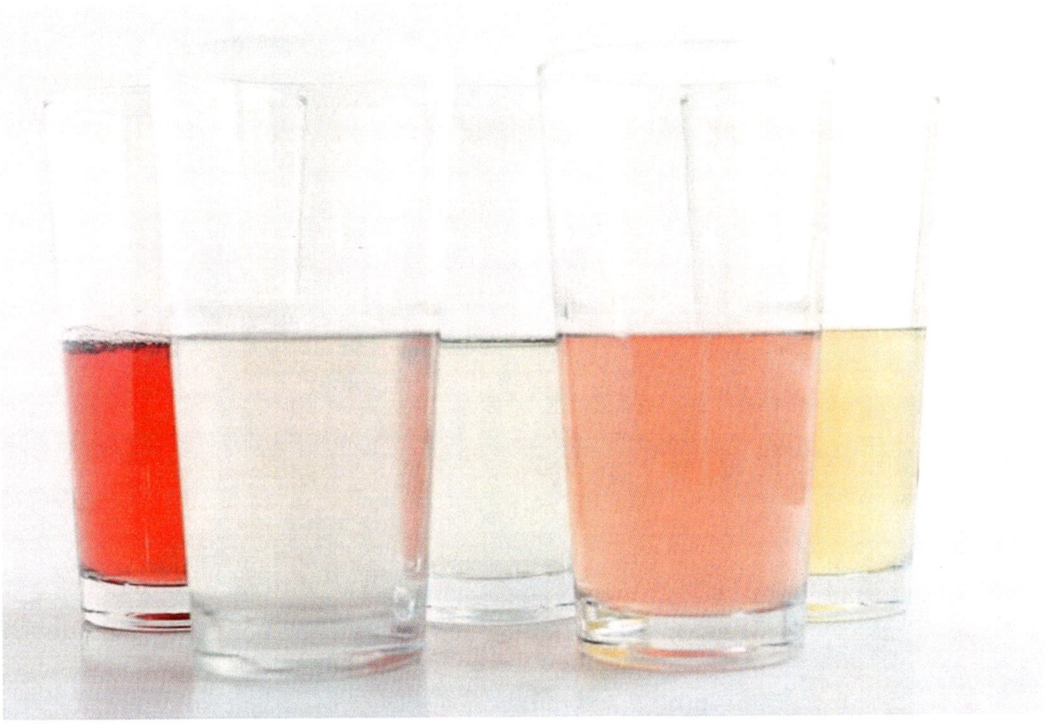

Prep Time: 5 minutes. Cook Time: 5 minutes. Total Time: 10 minutes.

Infused Water is everyone's favorite way of drinking water. Infused Water is a refreshing, healthy and perfect way of quenching your thirst any day of the year. Use the Instant Pot to extract every last bit of flavor from the fruits and vegetables you are infusing.

Servings: 4-5 cups

Ingredients

Apple-cinnamon

1 apple, chopped
2 cinnamon sticks

Blueberry-lime

1 cup blueberries
1 lime, juice and zest

Blueberry-orange

1 cup blueberries
1 orange, juice and zest

Cucumber-lime

1 cup cucumber, chopped
1 lime, juice and zest

Mango-ginger

1 cup mango, peeled and chopped
2 (1 inch) ginger knobs, peeled

Orange-basil

1 cup orange, thinly sliced and zest

5 large basil leaves

Peach-raspberry-lemonade

1 cup peaches, chopped
½ cup raspberries
1 lemon, juice and zest

Strawberry-mint

1 cup strawberries
½ cup mint leaves

Instructions

1. Place your choice of fruits, vegetables or herbs in a steam basket and place the steam basket in the Instant Pot.
2. Pour about 4-5 cups of water in the Instant Pot. Cover the lid and ensure the Pressure Release Valve is set to "Sealing."
3. Press the "Manual" Setting and cook at "High Pressure" for 5 minutes.
4. Once the timer goes off, do a Quick Pressure Release. Open the lid and carefully remove the steam basket. Discard the produce and set aside the liquid to cool.
5. Use as a concentrate or pour on ice cubes trays and freeze for later use.
6. Enjoy!

Green Tea

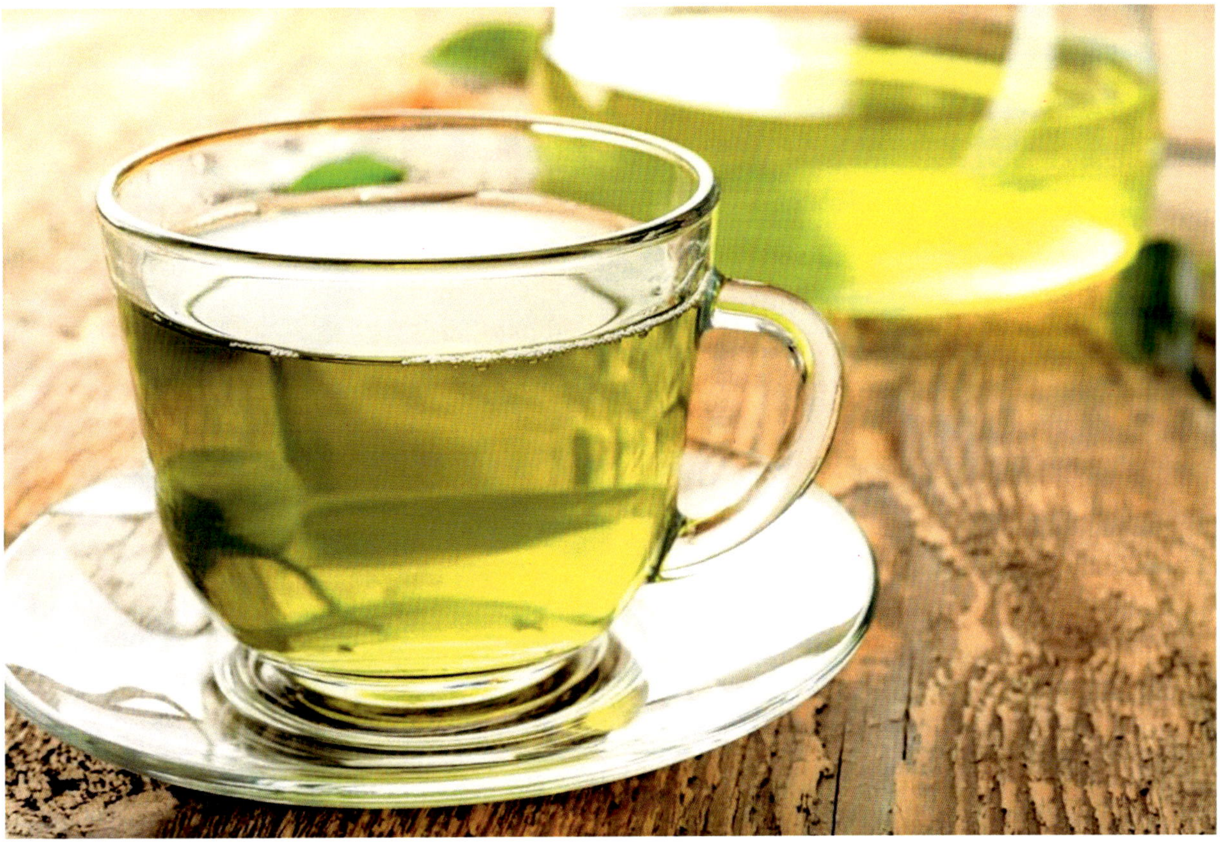

Prep Time: 5 minutes. Cook Time: 4 minutes. Total Time: 9 minutes.

Green tea is one of those drinks everyone orders in the coffee shop. If you are looking for healthy iced drinks to spruce up your afternoons, switch things up a little with the Instant Pot Green Tea.

Servings: 8

Ingredients

- 10 green tea bags
- 16 cups water
- 1/4 cup honey
- Basil leaves
- Lemon slices
- Lime slices

Optional

- 1 pinch baking soda

Instructions

1. Pour water into the Instant Pot and mix in baking soda and honey then stir until it dissolves.

2. Remove the tea bag tags and tie all the strings together so that it's easier to remove the tea bags.
3. Close the lid and ensure the Pressure Valve is turned to "Sealing." Set the Instant Pot to "Manual" setting and cook at "High Pressure" for 4 minutes.
4. Once cooked do a Quick Pressure Release. Let the tea sit a while. Pour the tea into a pitcher and cool in the refrigerator.
5. Serve hot or cold over ice with basil leaves, lime and lemon slices. Add more honey to sweeten the tea.

Iced Tea

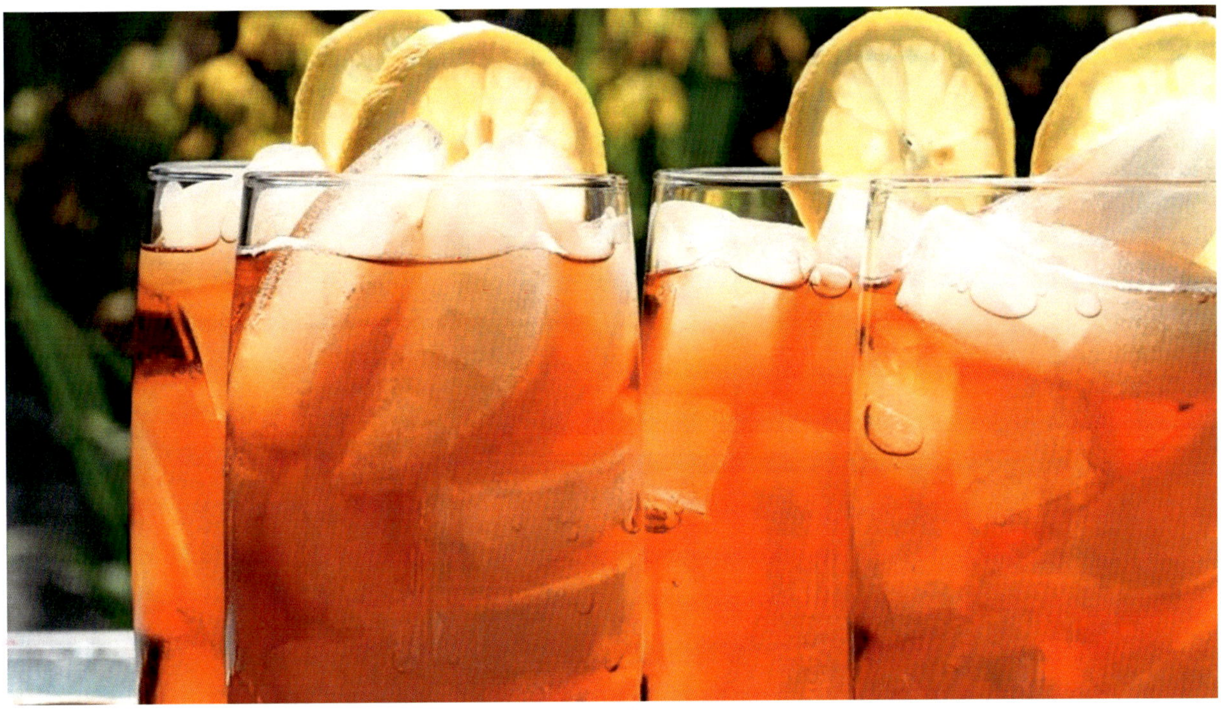

Prep Time: 10 minutes. Cook Time: 4 minutes. Total Time: 14 minutes.

Forget making Iced Tea the old fashion way, enjoy a strong yet mellow glass of Instant Pot iced tea. Instant Pot provides an easy and hands-off method for this flavorful and refreshing drink.

Servings: 8.

Ingredients

4 regular tea bags, tag-less or remove the tag
6 cups water
½ cup sugar

Instructions

1. Pour 6 cups of water in the Instant Pot, add the sugar and place in the teabags.
2. Seal the lid. Program the Instant Pot to "Manual" setting with a 4-minute preparation time length and cook on "High Pressure."
3. Allow Natural Pressure Release for about 10-15 minutes then carefully open the lid.
4. Set aside to cool then serve over ice.
5. Enjoy!

Wassail

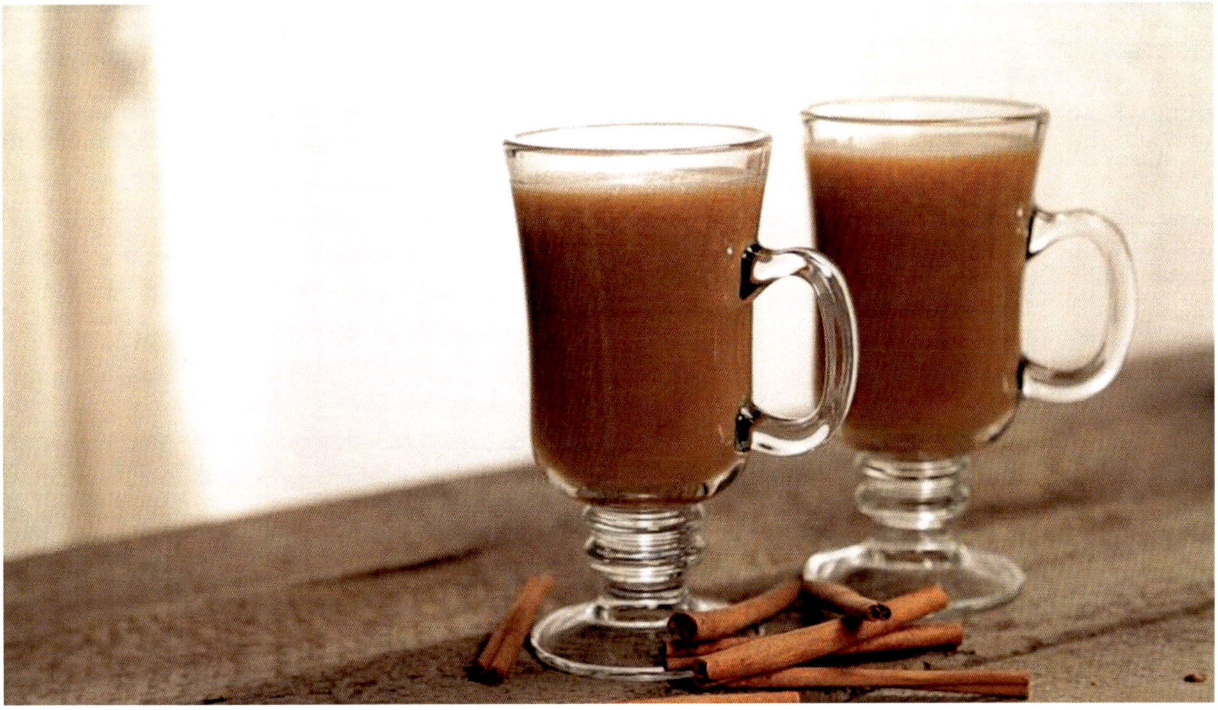

Prep Time: 5 minutes. Cook Time: 10 minutes. Total Time: 15 minutes.

Wassail is a popular winter and fall season drink. The warm, naturally sweetened steamy drink is the ultimate culmination of wonderful autumn smells. This drink is sure to bring back sweet childhood memories.

Servings: 12 cups

Ingredients

8 cups apple cider
4 cups orange juice
2 lemons, juice and zest
10 cloves
5 cinnamon sticks
2 vanilla beans, split
1-inch ginger, peeled
½ teaspoon nutmeg, freshly grated

Instructions

1. Pour the apple cider and orange juice into the Instant Pot. Place the steam basket into the Instant Pot then add vanilla beans, cinnamon sticks, nutmeg, cloves, ginger, lemon juice and zest.
2. Close the lid and ensure the Pressure Releasing Valve is set to "Sealing" position.
3. Set the Instant Pot to "Manual" setting and cook at "High Pressure" and cook for 10 minutes.

4. When the timer goes off, allow Natural Pressure Release for about 10 minutes.
5. Carefully open the lid and remove the steam basket the discard the contents of the steamer basket.
6. Serve the wassail hot.
7. Enjoy!

Cough Syrup

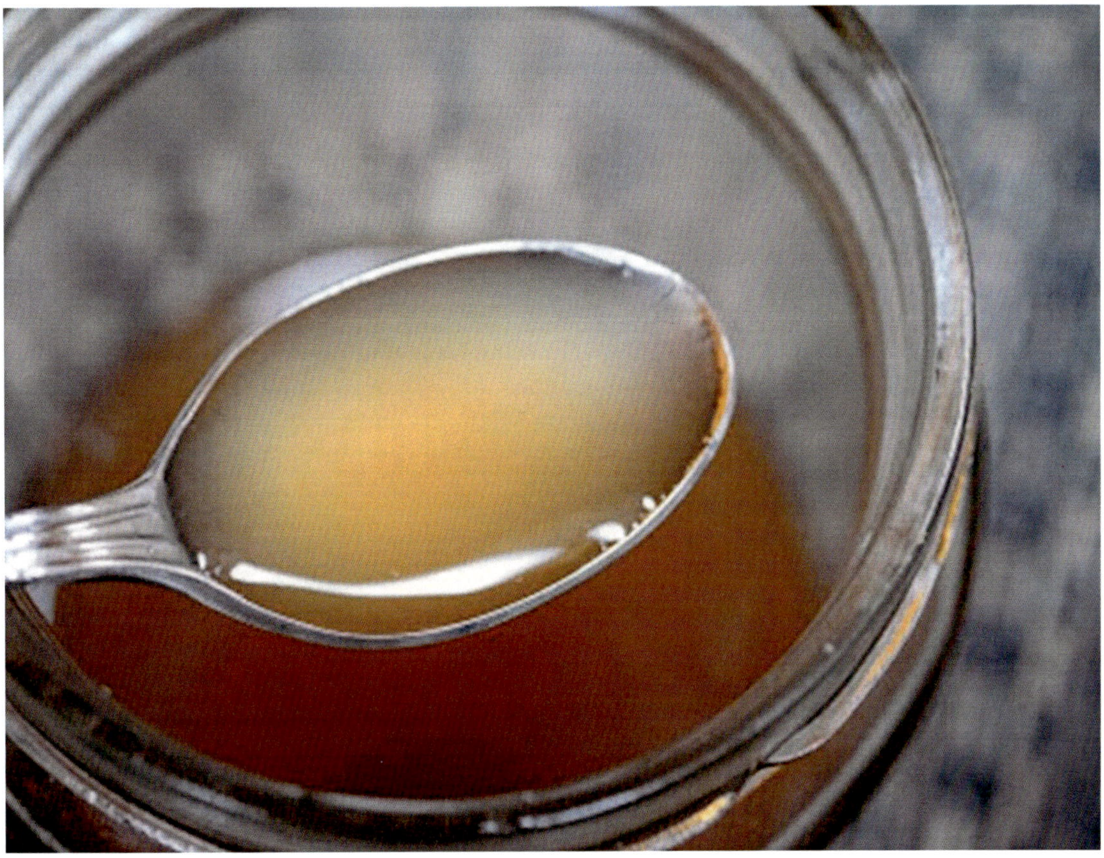

Prep Time: 5 minutes. Cook Time: 10 minutes. Total Time: 15 minutes.

Medicine cabinets are always filled with cough and cold prescription bottles as well as other over the counter medication. It's no harm to switch these up with homemade cures that actually work. The Instant Pot Cold Syrup is made of cheap and readily available ingredients. Store the cough syrup in the refrigerator for 1-2 months.

Servings: use whenever you get a cough.

Ingredients

2 cups water
¼ cup raw honey
¼ cup fresh ginger, chopped into small pieces
¼ cup thyme sprigs
1 lemon, juiced
¼ teaspoon cayenne pepper

Instructions

1. Pour water into the Instant Pot then add thyme and ginger.
2. Program the Instant Pot to "Sauté" function and cook for 10 minutes until the liquid in the pot is reduced to about half.

3. Cancel the "sauté" function and let the mixture cool. Strain the mixture and discard the chopped ginger and thyme sprigs.
4. Stir in cayenne pepper, raw honey, and lemon juice.
5. Pour the mixed cough syrup into an airtight storage container and leave in the refrigerator.
6. Get well soon!

FRUITS AND VEGETABLES

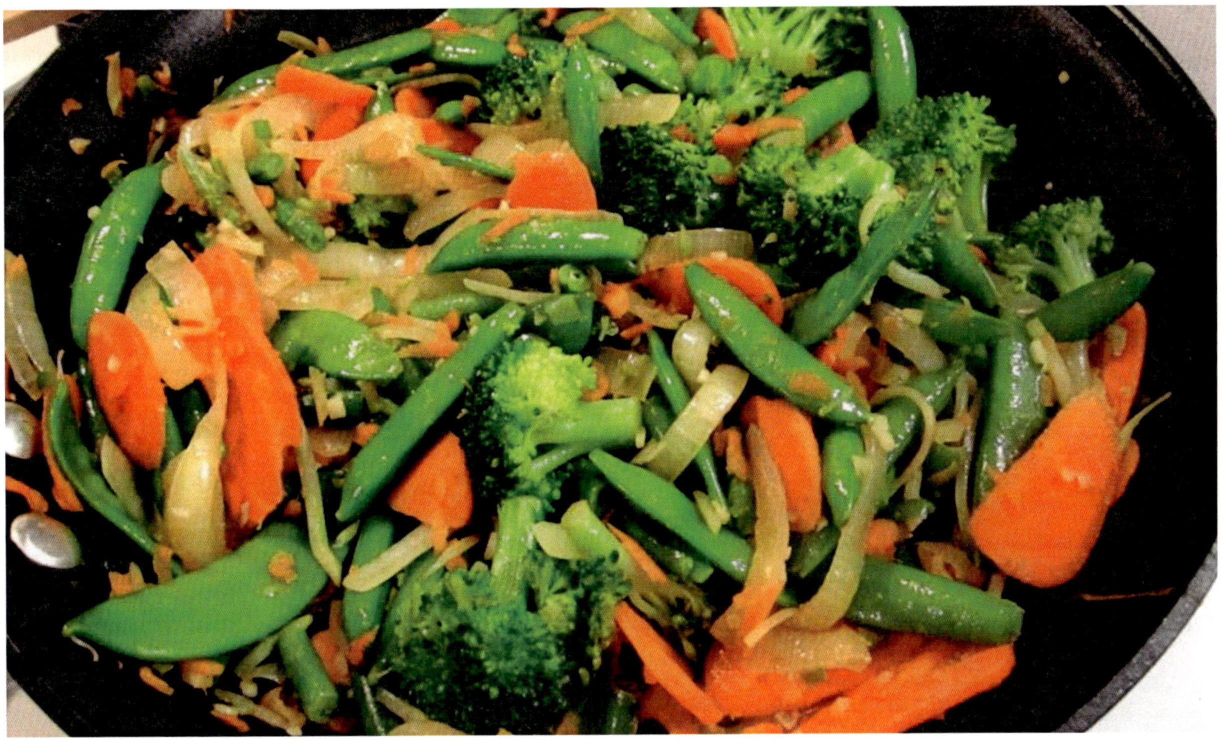

Different beautiful colors are nature's way of proving that fruits and vegetables are good for us. Make every meal unforgettable with fruits and veggies. If you are a picky eater, then you probably don't eat enough fruits and veggies. Use the ever-expanding collection of tasty, delicious and tantalizing Instant Pot fruits and vegetable recipes to work more fruits and veggies into your diet. You can easily make vegetable and fruit dishes with an Instant Pot, and we have made it easy with these great inspirations. These recipes perfectly blend and tie together different textures and fresh hue of fruits and vegetables. The recipes below full of nutrients and flavors, so pick a few and try them out.

Blueberry Jam

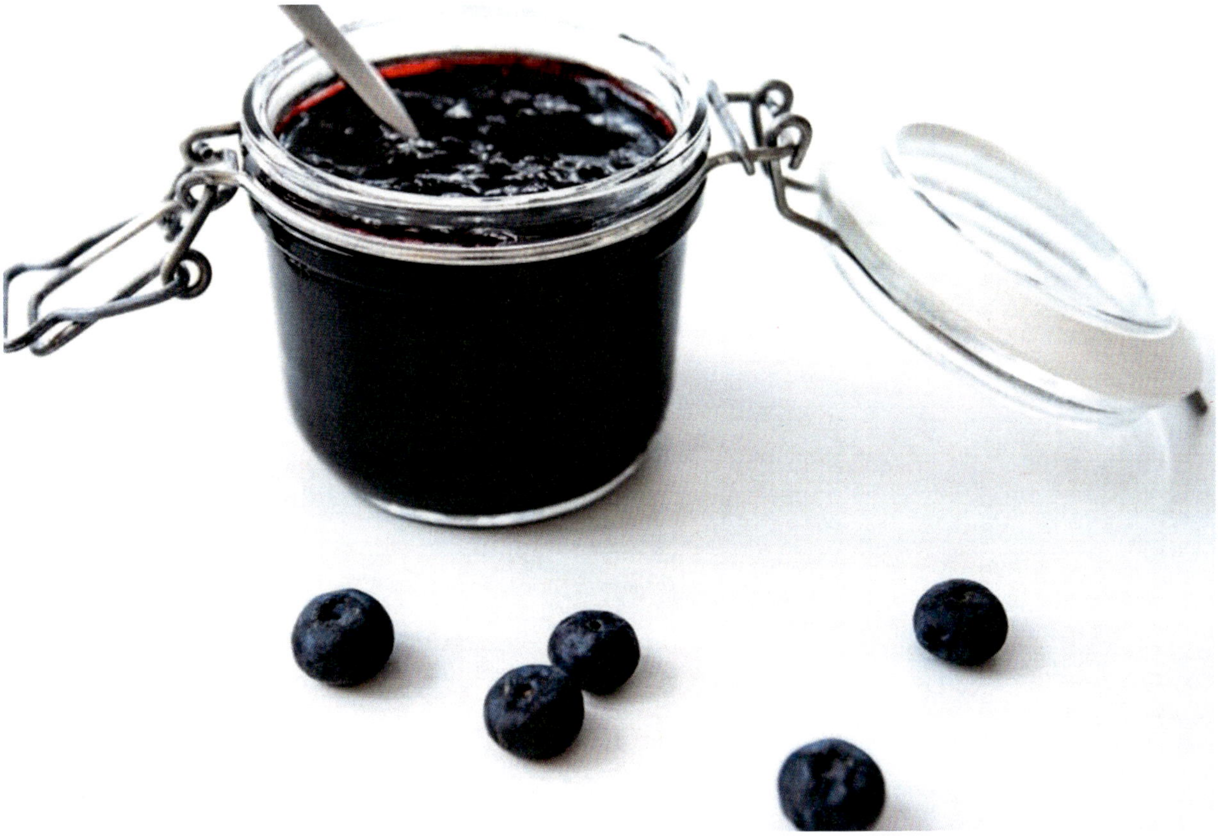

Prep Time: 10 minutes. Cook Time: 18 minutes. Total Time: 28 minutes.

If you love Blueberry Jam as much as I do, then you know how easy it is to go through jars. Save extra bucks by making healthy and tasty Blueberry Jam in the Instant Pot.

Servings: 2-pint size jars

Ingredients

1 lb fresh or frozen blueberries
½ lb sugar
1 lemon, juice and zest

Instructions

1. If you are using frozen blueberries thaw first, place them in a food processor or blender and puree.
2. Add sugar and mix well. You can add more sugar if you find the mixture tart.
3. To make a perfect blend refrigerate the mixture.
4. After refrigeration, add the lemon zest and lemon juice into the mixture.
5. Stir the mixture and pour into the Instant Pot. Program the Instant Pot to the "Sauté" function bring the blueberry and lemon mixture to a boil for about 5 minutes.
6. Cancel the "Sauté" function and seal the lid. Set the Instant Pot to "Manual" function and cook on "High Pressure" for 5 minutes.

7. Allow Nature Pressure Release when the timer goes off and open the lid carefully. Reset the Instant Pot to "Sauté" function and bring back the jam to a boil. Stir constantly for 5 minutes and set aside to cool.
8. Once cooled freeze or refrigerate the jam for later.
9. Enjoy!

Strawberry Jam

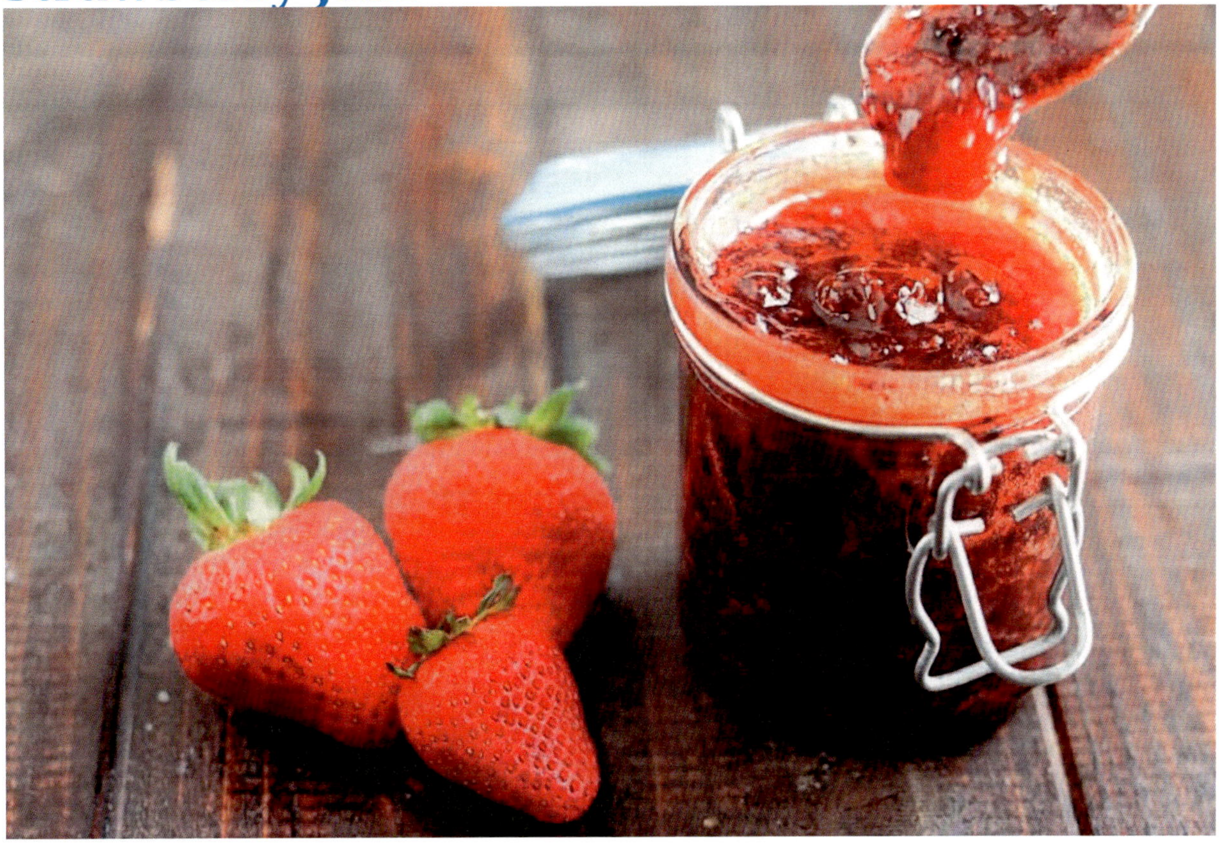

Prep Time: 5 minutes. Cook Time: 10 minutes. Total Time: 15 minutes.

It's amazing how quick and easy it is to make homemade jam. This tasty organic Strawberry Jam is healthy and kid-friendly with no preservatives. The best part you don't have to worry about burning the jam mid-cook.

Servings: 2-pint size jars

Ingredients

1 lb organic strawberries, diced
1 cup raw honey

Instructions

1. Set the Instant Pot to "Sauté" function then pour in the honey. Melt the honey until you can easily stir it before adding the strawberries.
2. Bring the strawberries to a boil and let them simmer for about 3-4 minutes then close the lid. Ensure the Pressure Release Valve is set to "Sealing" position.
3. Cancel the "Sauté" function. Program the Instant Pot to "Manual" and cook on "High Pressure" for 3 minutes.
4. Once the timer goes off, allow Natural Pressure Release then carefully open the lid. Mash or use a hand blender to puree the mixture.

5. Reset the instant Pot to "Sauté" function and bring the strawberry jam to a boil. The jam will coat the back of a spoon when ready.
6. Remove the jam from heat and set aside to cool
7. Pour the strawberry jam into an airtight container and store in the refrigerator for later.
8. Enjoy!

Cranberry Sauce

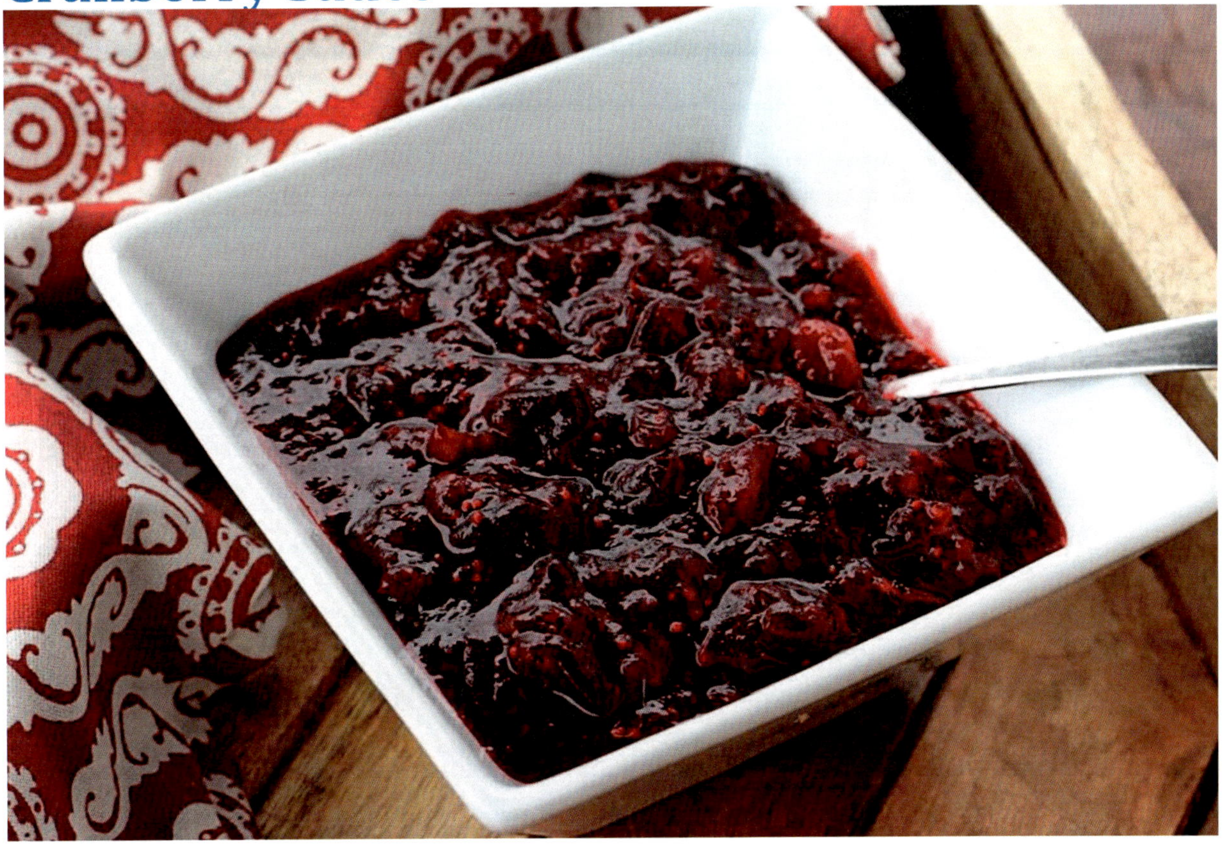

Prep Time: 15 minutes. Cook Time: 1 minute. Total Time: 16 minutes.

The tangy-sweet Instant Pot Cranberry Sauce is a great jam-like spread that can also be used as filling for pastries, topping for desserts, extra flavor for smoothie/ yogurt or glaze for meat. Make Cranberry Sauce a whole year affair instead of only saving it for Thanksgiving and Christmas dinner.

Servings: 1 cup

Ingredients

12 oz cranberries
½ - 1 cup white sugar
¼ cup freshly squeezed orange
2 ½ teaspoons orange zest
1 pinch salt

Optional

2 tablespoons honey or maple syrup

Instructions

1. Pour the orange juice and add the 10oz cranberries, orange zest, honey or maple syrup. Reserve 2oz cranberries for later.

2. Seal the lid and set the Instant Pot to "Manual" setting and cook at "High Pressure" for 1 minute.
3. When the timer goes off, allow Natural Pressure Release for about 7 minutes before carefully opening the lid.
4. Click "Cancel" then reset the Instant Pot to "Sauté" function. Use a wooden spoon to stir the mixture. Add in Sugar and the remaining cranberries. Stir to melt the sugar. Add a pinch of salt and any additional sugar if desired.
5. Serve warm or cold with your favorite dish.
6. Enjoy!

Blueberry Compote

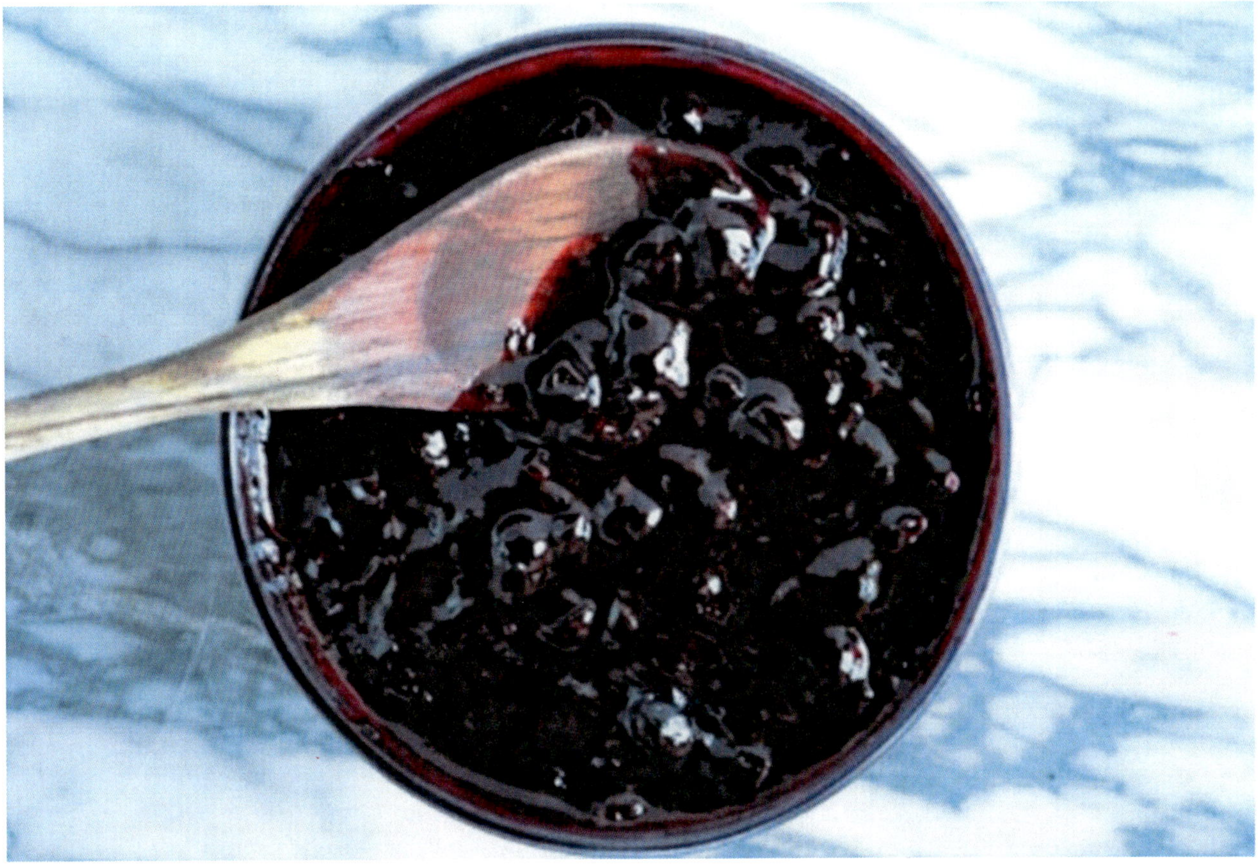

Prep Time: 10 minutes. Cook Time: 5 minutes. Total Time: 15 minutes.

Learn how to easily and quickly make yummy Blueberry Compote in your Instant Pot. This 5-ingredient homemade goodness is a great cheesecake, dessert, yogurt and breakfast topping. Adjust this recipe to make a strawberry compote.

Servings: 1 cup

Ingredients

1 lb blueberries
2 tablespoons white sugar or maple syrup
2 tablespoons freshly squeezed lemon juice
1 teaspoon lemon zest
½ teaspoon cinnamon powder
1 pinch salt

Instructions

1. Reserve some blueberries (1/3) for texture then place the remaining blueberries into the Instant Pot. Add in the lemon juice, lemon zest, cinnamon powder, and salt.

2. Seal the lid. Program the Instant Pot to "Manual" setting and cook on "High Pressure" for 1 minute. Once the timer goes off, allow Natural Pressure Release for about 10 minutes. Carefully open the lid.
3. Click the "Cancel" button then set the Instant Pot to "Sauté" function and turn to "Medium Heat." Use a wooden spoon to stir and break the berries then add in the remaining blueberries. Add the white sugar or maple syrup and stir to thicken the blueberry compote. Add more sweetener if desired.
4. Chill and pour into an airtight container. Store the blueberry compote for 10-12 days in the refrigerator.

Instant Pot Applesauce

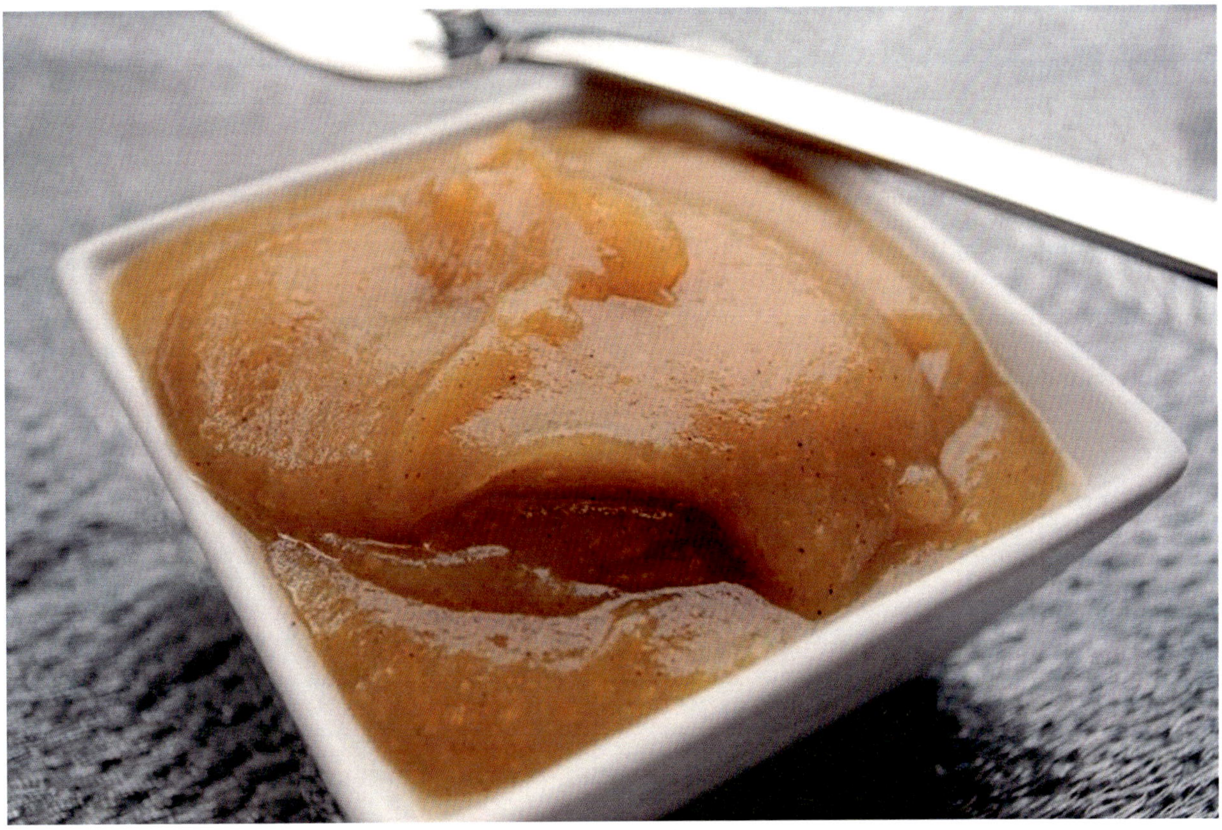

Prep Time: 10 minutes. Cook Time: 5 minutes. Total Time: 15 minutes.

Everyone loves the warm and comforting smell of cinnamon and apples drifting from the kitchen. Homemade Applesauce is about to become your new family tradition. The cinnamon spiced apple treat is quite flavorful with a perfect balance of sweet, savory and slightly tart. The thick apple puree is delicious as a filling, topping, condiment or dessert.

Servings: 800ml.

Ingredients

3 lbs apples, quartered
¼ cup water
1-2 cinnamon sticks
¼ - ½ teaspoon nutmeg
1 pinch salt
Honey to taste

Instructions

1. Pour water into the Instant Pot then add in the quartered apples, cinnamon sticks, and nutmeg.
2. Seal the lid. Set the Instant Pot to "Manual" function and cook at "High Pressure" for 5 minutes.

3. Allow Natural Pressure Release then carefully open the lid.
4. Remove the cinnamon sticks and discard. Puree the mixture in a blender. Add a pinch of salt and honey to taste.
5. Cool and store in the refrigerator for later use.

Stuffed Peaches

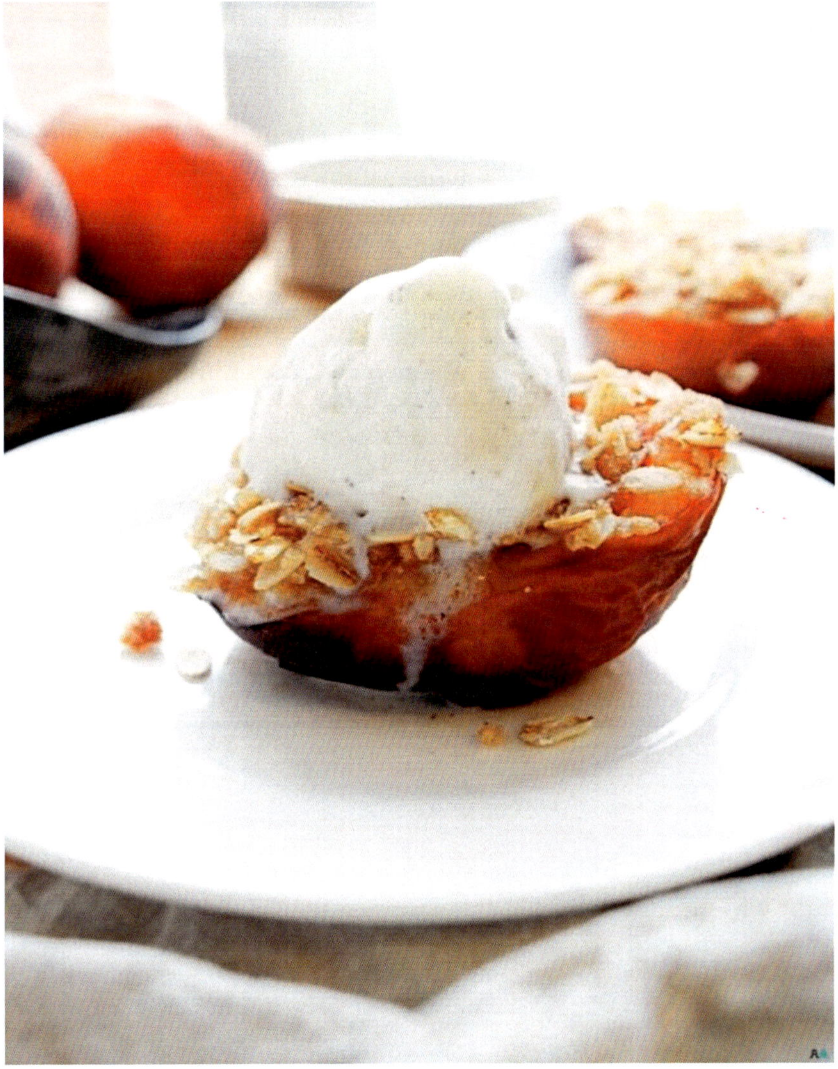

Prep Time: 15 minutes. Cook Time: 3 minutes. Total Time: 18 minutes.

Each bite of this fresh summer treat feels like it's truly something special and refreshing. Peaches are great summer fruits. They are sweet, juicy and taste heavenly in baked goodies. The Instant Pot Stuffed Peaches are pure goodness with the cinnamon cobbler stuffing and ice cream topping. If you love a peach pie, this easy-to-make treat tastes just like it, making them a fun afternoon snack.

Servings: 5

Ingredients

- 5 medium peaches
- 1 cup water
- ¼ cup sugar
- ¼ cup flour
- 2 tablespoon butter
- 2¼ teaspoon pure almond extract

½ teaspoon ground cinnamon
1 pinch sea salt

Instructions

1. Slice off ¼ inch tops of the peaches and discard. Use a sharp paring knife or a spoon to cut around, remove and scoop the pits. Set aside the hollowed-out peaches.
2. In a mixing bowl and flour and sweetener of choice, almond extract, cinnamon, butter and sea salt. Use your hands to combine the ingredients into a crumbly mixture.
3. Fill and top the peaches with the crumble mixture.
4. Pour water into the Instant Pot and add in ¼ teaspoon almond extract. Put a steamer basket into the pot and carefully place the stuffed peaches on top of it.
5. Close the lid and ensure the Steam Release Valve is set to "Sealing" position.
6. Program the Instant Pot to "Manual" mode and set the timer for 3 minutes. Once the timer beeps do a Quick Pressure Release then carefully open the lid. Remove the steamer basket and place the stuffed peaches on serving plate. Set aside to cool.
7. Serve topped with vanilla ice cream.
8. Enjoy!

Vegetable Stock

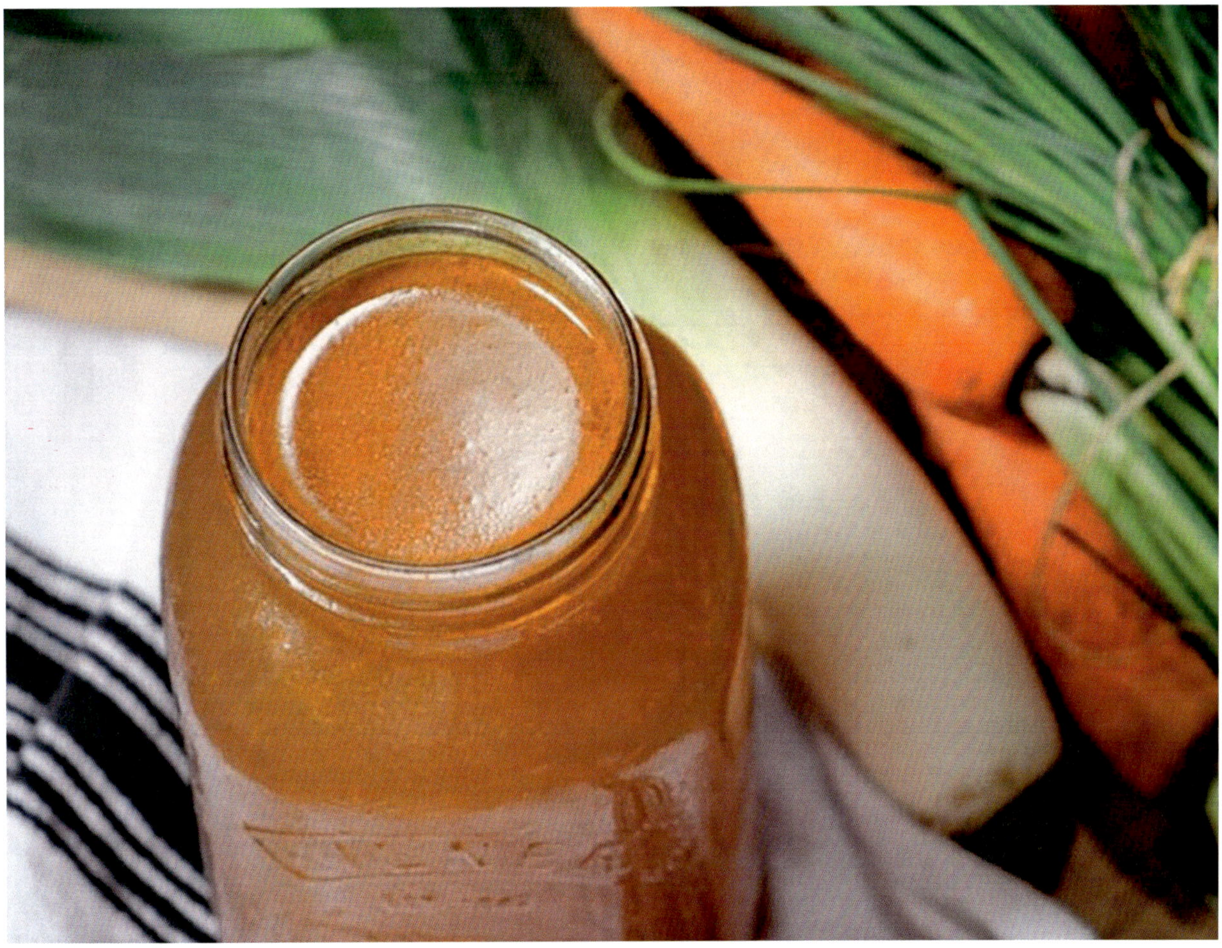

Prep Time: 5 minutes. Cook Time: 15 minutes. Total Time: 20 minutes.

A good stock is a kitchen's staple and an essential ingredient to enhance any dish. Add extra depth to the flavors and texture to your soups, sauces or other dishes with this homemade vegetable stock. This Instant Pot Vegetable Stock recipe is a healthier alternative to the store-bought stock. Make this nourishing Vegetable Stock with your leftover veggies.

Servings: 1 jar.

Ingredients

2 small onions, roughly chopped
6 cremini mushrooms, roughly sliced
1 Shiitake mushroom, dried
4 cloves garlic, crushed
6 carrots, roughly diced
2 celery stalks, roughly diced
2 bay leaves
8 cups water
2 tablespoons light soy sauce

1 teaspoon peppercorn

Instructions

1. Place all the ingredients in the Instant Pot and close the lid.
2. Program the Instant Pot to "Manual" function and cook at "High Pressure" for 15 minutes.
3. Allow Natural Pressure Release when the timer goes off for about 15 minutes. Then turn the Pressure Release Valve to "Venting" position.
4. Carefully open the lid. Use a fine-mesh strainer to strain the stock. Set the vegetable stock aside to cool.
5. Refrigerate or freeze the veggie stock for later. If refrigerated the stock lasts for about 5-7 days and 2-3 months if frozen.

Spaghetti Squash

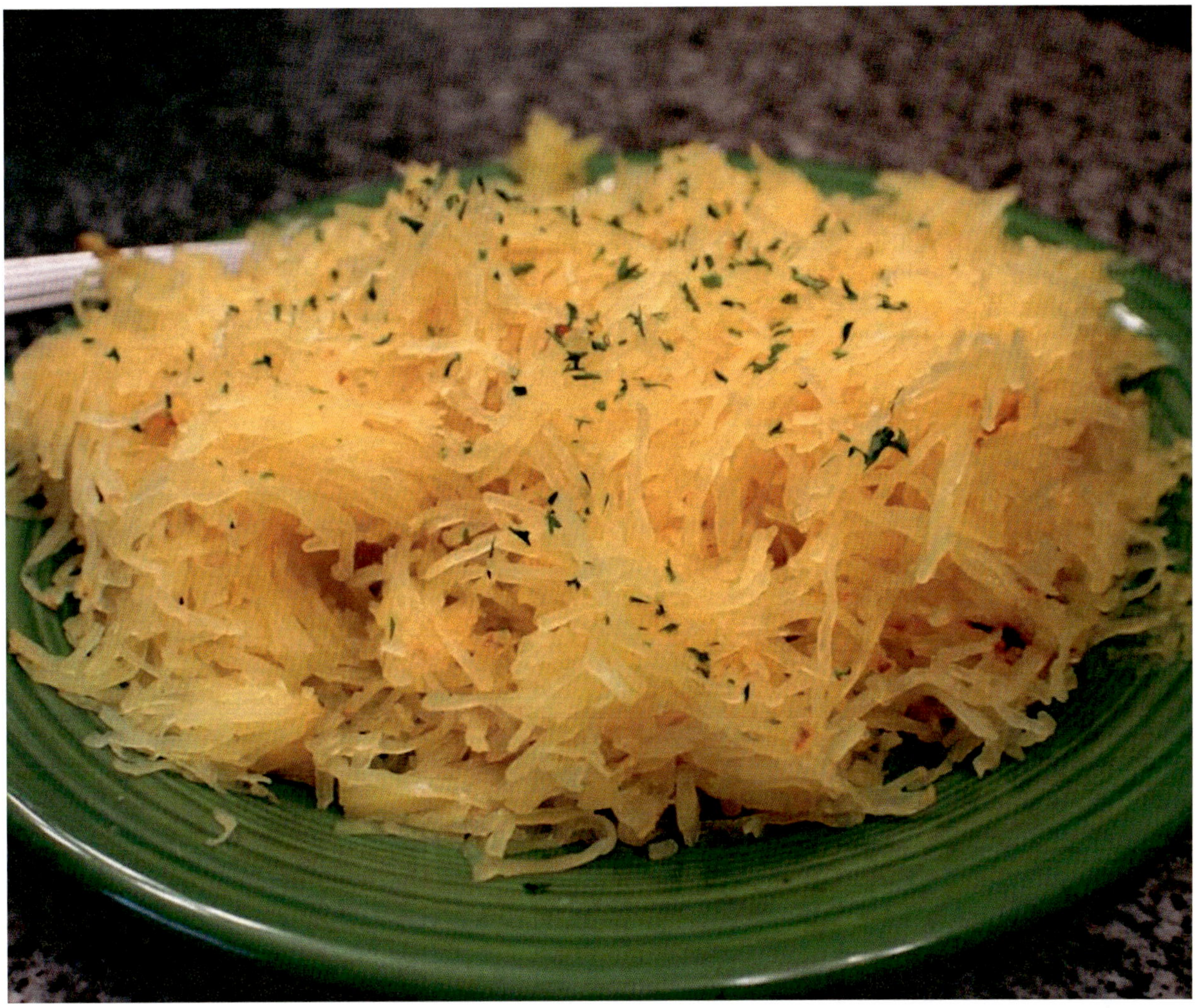

Prep Time: 10 minutes. Cook Time: 6-8 minutes. Total Time: 16-18 minutes.

When fully cooked the spaghetti squash creates thin translucent strands that can easily substitute pasta. The Instant Pot Spaghetti Squash has a mild, delicate flavor, watery structure, and a refreshing light crunch. Spaghetti squash is suitable for low-carb, gluten-free and Paleo diets and serves great as a no-fuss noodly guiltless treat or a healthy salad

Servings: 2-4.

Ingredients

1 whole spaghetti squash
1 cup water

Instructions

1. Use a sharp knife to the spaghetti squash in half, lengthwise. The use a spoon to scoop out the seeds and scrape the bits.

2. Pour water into the Instant Pot and Place a trivet in the pot. Carefully the spaghetti squash on the trivet. Close the lid.
3. Set the Instant Pot to "Manual" setting and "High Pressure." For al dente spaghetti squash set the timer for 6 minutes and for softer spaghetti squash set the cook timer for 8 minutes.
4. When the timer goes off, do a Quick Pressure Release then carefully open the lid.
5. Remove the spaghetti squash from the Instant Pot. Use a fork to gently pull the flesh creating "spaghetti-like" strands.
6. Serve hot and enjoy!

Herbed Potatoes

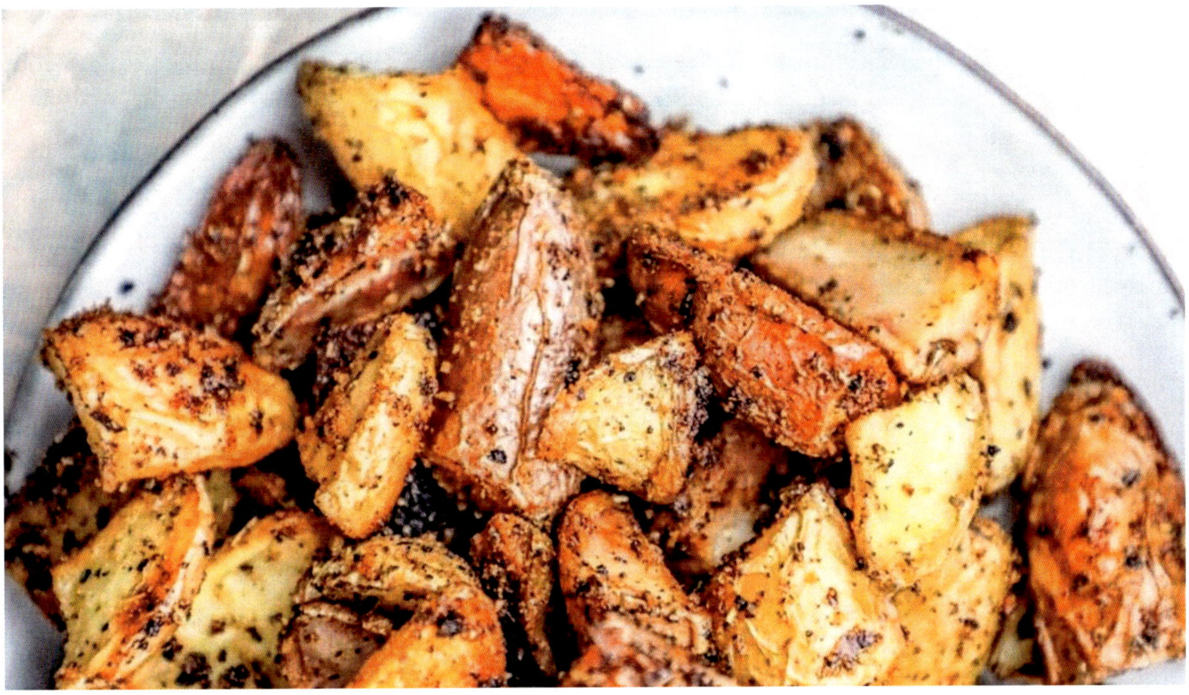

Prep Time: 5 minutes. Cook Time: 5 minutes. Total Time: 10 minutes.

You probably have potatoes in the pantry, and you don't need to go to the store for other ingredients. Instant Pot Herbed Potatoes are delicious and easy to make veggie snack dish.

Servings: 2-4.

Ingredients

6-8 potatoes, roughly diced
¼ small onion, minced
¼ cup water
4 tablespoons butter
1 tablespoon fresh parsley, chopped
1 teaspoon garlic, minced
1 teaspoon Italian seasoning
½ teaspoon dried dill
Salt and pepper to taste

Instructions

1. Pour water into the Instant Pot then place in the potatoes. Stir in the other ingredients and drop the butter on top in dollops.
2. Seal the lid. Program the Instant Pot to "Stew" and cook for 5 minutes.
3. Allow Natural Pressure Release when the timer goes off this might take 10 minutes. Carefully open the lid. For crispy potatoes drain the liquid, add

more butter then program the Instant Pot to "Sauté" function. Cook for approximately 8 minutes until the potatoes are browned.

4. Taste and adjust seasoning then serve hot.
5. Enjoy!

Instant Pot Brussels Sprouts

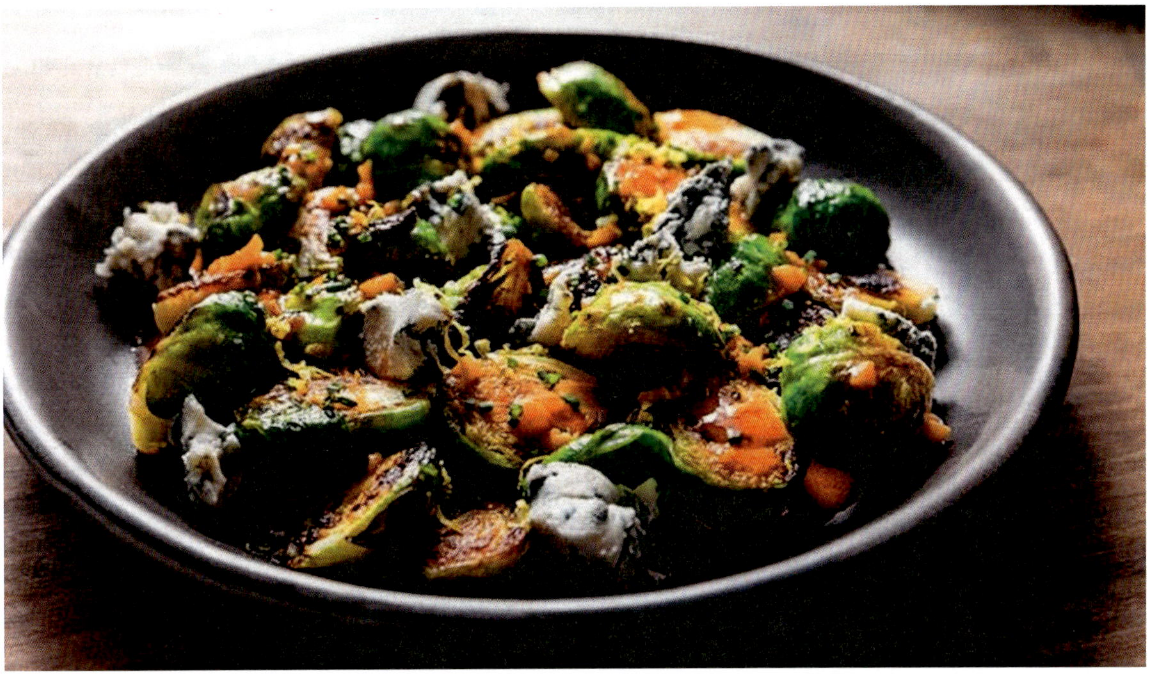

Prep Time: 5 minutes. Cook Time: 3 minutes. Total Time: 8 minutes.

Feels like Brussels Sprouts are fairly underrated when it comes to vegetables. Most people set them aside but if cooked right Brussel Sprouts are absolutely amazing. The Instant Pot Brussels Sprouts recipe does just that.

Servings: 6-8.

Ingredients

2 lbs Brussels sprouts, halved
¼ cup soy sauce
2 tablespoons sesame oil
2 tablespoons sriracha sauce
1 tablespoon almonds, chopped
1 tablespoon rice vinegar
1 teaspoon onion powder
2 teaspoons garlic powder
1 teaspoon smoked paprika
1 teaspoon red pepper flakes
½ teaspoon cayenne pepper
Salt and pepper to taste

Instructions

1. Program the Instant Pot to "Sauté" function and put the almonds in the pot. Mix in all your seasonings and liquids into the Instant Pot.
2. Add the halved Brussels sprouts, stir and close the lid.

3. Click the "Cancel" button and set the Instant Pot to "Manual" function and cook at "High Pressure" for 3 minutes.
4. When the timer goes off, do a Quick Pressure Release and carefully open the lid.
5. Serve and enjoy!

Orange Spiced Carrots

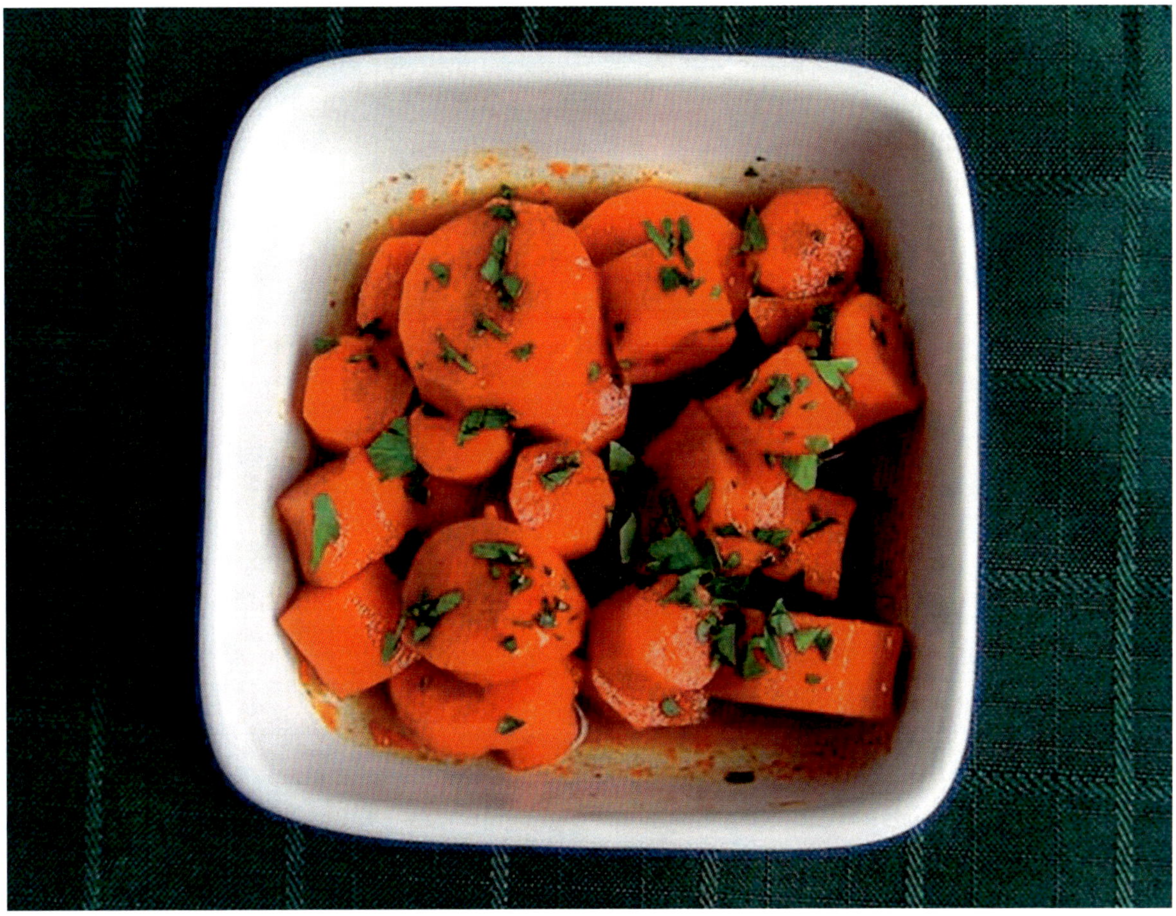

Prep Time: 10 minutes. Cook Time: 5 minutes. Total Time: 15 minutes.

Orange Spiced Carrots mix and matches spices and flavors for a tantalizing veggie meal. This recipe is kid friendly and a great way to get your kids to eat vegetables. Top Orange Spiced Carrots with orange zest to add that extra zing.

Servings: 6.

Ingredients

2 lbs baby carrots or medium carrots, cut into 1 inch
¼ cup water
½ cup orange juice
½ cup brown sugar
1 tablespoon cornstarch
2 tablespoons butter
¼ teaspoon ground nutmeg
¾ teaspoon ground cinnamon
½ teaspoon salt

Instructions

1. Place all the ingredients except water and cornstarch in the Instant Pot. Close the lid and ensure the Pressure Release Vent is set to "Sealing" position.
2. Program the Instant Pot to "Manual" setting and cook at "Low pressure" for 3 minutes.
3. Once the timer goes off, do a Quick Pressure Release carefully open the lid and cancel "Manual" setting.
4. Set the Instant Pot to "Sauté" setting and adjust for to cook at "High Pressure." Add water and cornstarch in a small bowl and mix until smooth. Stir in this combination into the carrot mixture. Gradually stir and let the mixture cook to a thicken sauce for about 1-2 minutes.
5. Serve and enjoy!

Instant Pot Beets

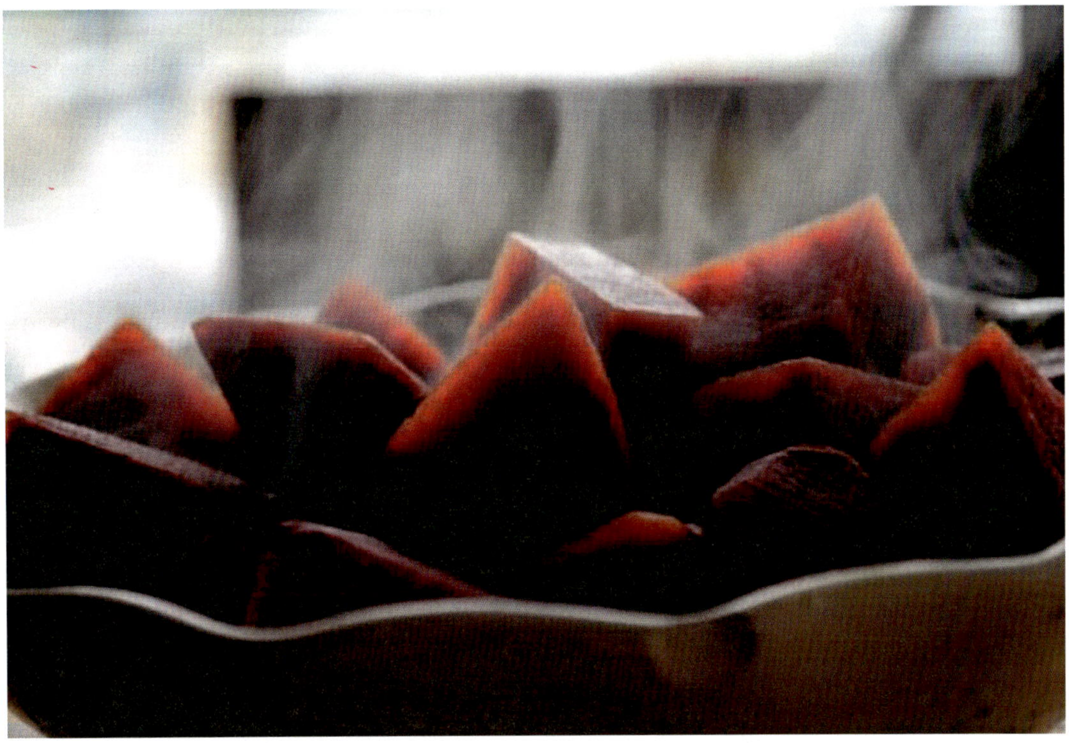

Prep Time: 5 minutes. Cook Time: 25 minutes. Total Time: 30 minutes.

Beets are healthy and nutritious. They are great additives to smoothies, salads, purees, desserts and pickled snacks. You are going to enjoy the refreshing crunch of these Instant Pot beets. They are juicy, sweet and chewy. Kids are going to enjoy playing around with fake blood-stained fingers and tongues from eating the beets.

Servings: 6

Ingredients

6 medium beets
1 cup water

Instructions

1. Thoroughly wash the beets then trim off and discard the roots, stems, and greens.
2. Pour 1 cup of water into the Instant Pot and place a steam basket in the pot. Place the beets in the steam basket and close the lid.
3. Program the Instant Pot to cook at "High Pressure" for 25 minutes.
4. Do a Quick Pressure Release when the cook time lapses and carefully open the lid.
5. You can either peel the beets or leave the skin on as the skins are edible. Cut the beets into cubes and transfer into serving plates.
6. If desired season with salt. Serve hot or cold.
7. Enjoy!

Corn on the Cob

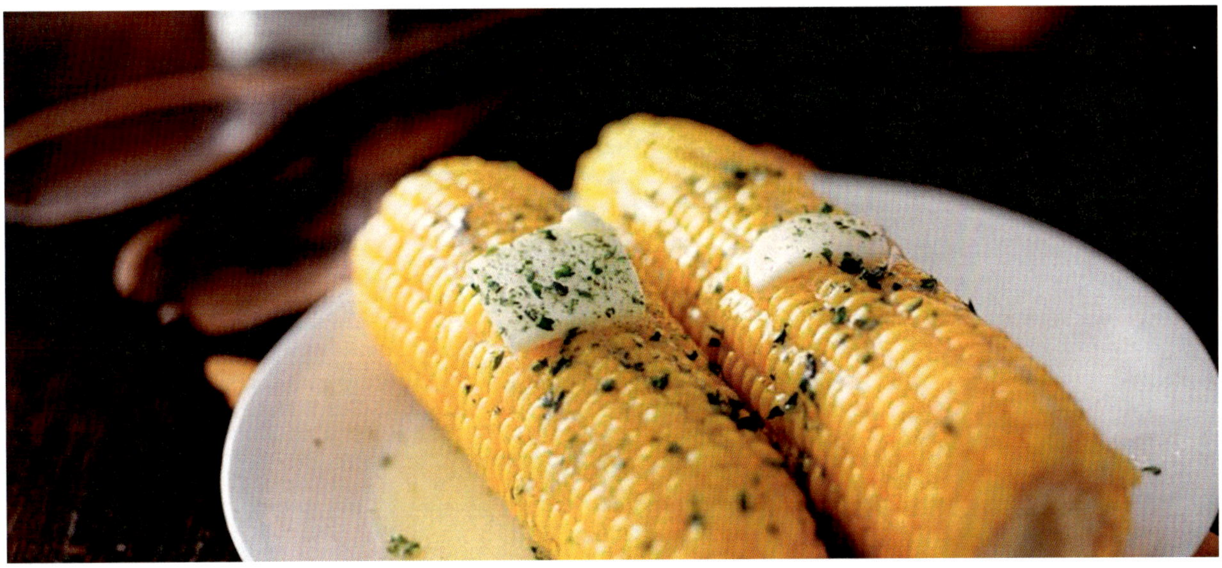

Prep Time: 5 minutes. Cook Time: 1 minute. Total Time: 6 minutes.

Corn on the Cob is an easy and quick to make fresh summer treat. Use an Instant Pot to make this healthy and family-friendly comfort food perfectly tender and juicy. Cooking corn on the cob in an Instant Pot maximizes nutrient retention as compared to the traditional cooking methods making it a great side dish.

Servings: 4

Ingredients

4 ears corn on the cob, silk and husks removed.
1 cup water.

Instructions

1. Pour 1 cup of water in the Instant Pot. Place the steam rack or a steam basket in the Instant Pot.
2. Place the corn on the steam rack or steam basket then seal the lid.
3. Set the Instant Pot to cook at "High Pressure" for 1-2 minutes.
4. Quick Release when the timer goes off and carefully open the lid.
5. Immediately serve with butter, your favorite corn toppings or sauce.
6. Enjoy!

Bacon Ranch Potatoes

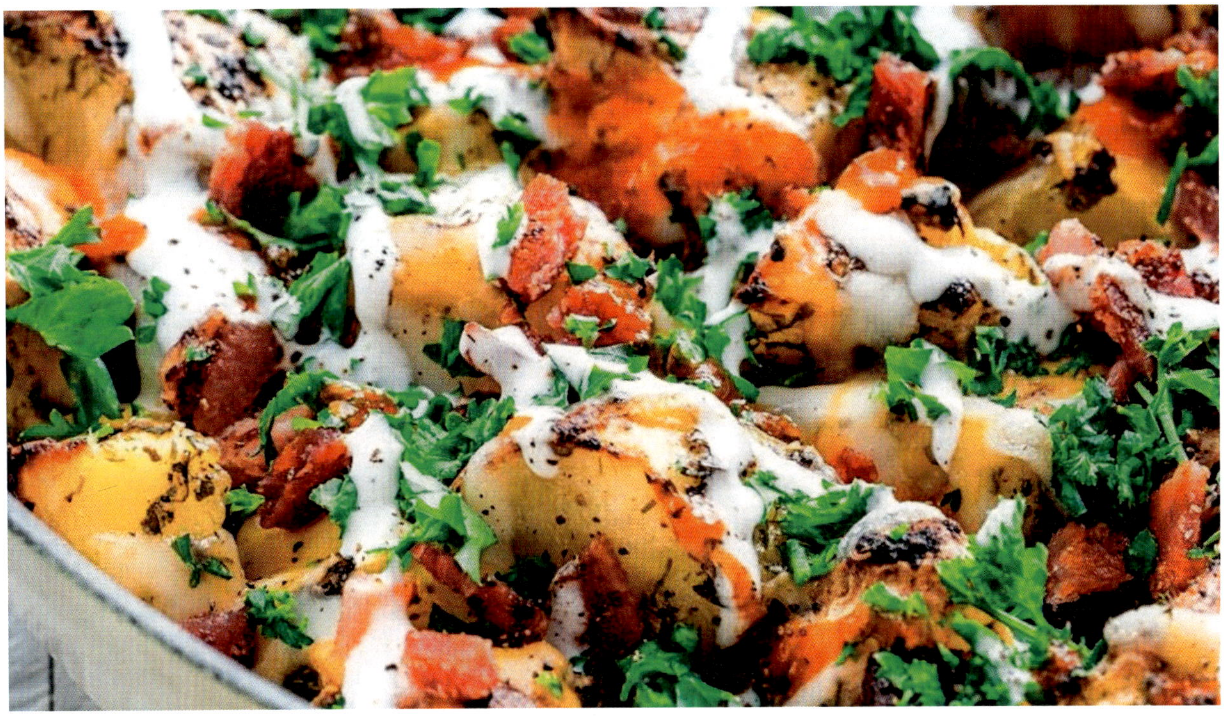

Prep Time: 10 minutes. Cook Time: 7-10 minutes. Total Time: 20 minutes.

With only 4 main ingredients and 3 simple seasonings, Bacon Ranch Potatoes is yet another easy-to-make Instant Pot tasty and mouth-watering comfort breakfast meal.

Servings: 6

Ingredients

2 lb scrubbed, Red Potatoes
4 oz Cheddar Cheese, shredded
3 Bacon Strips
1/3 cup Ranch Dressing
2 teaspoons Dried Parsley
1 teaspoon Garlic Powder
1 teaspoon Kosher Salt

Instructions

1. Dice the potatoes into 1-inch pieces.
2. Cut the bacon strips into smaller pieces.
3. Place the potato and bacon pieces into the Instant Pot then add 2 tablespoons of water. Stir in the salt, dried and garlic powder.
4. Program your Instant Pot to the "Manual" function and set the timer for 7 minutes (the cooking time varies with the size of the Instant Pot). Quick Release the pressure after the timer goes off then carefully open the lid.
5. Add some cheese and ranch dressing.
6. Serve immediately.

7. Enjoy!

ABOUT THE AUTHOR

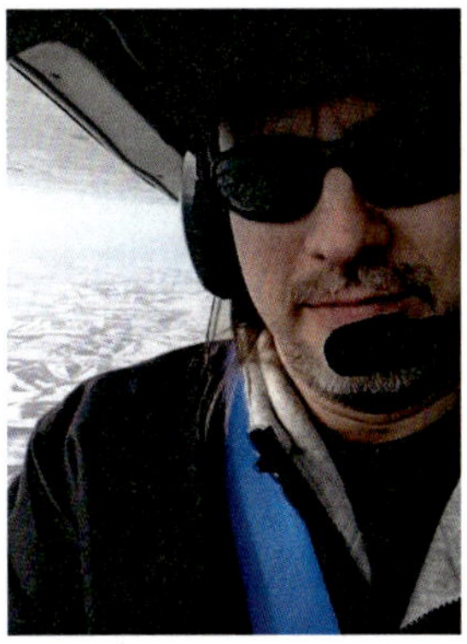

Born in Wichita Falls, Texas, Joe Boardman has traveled the world filling many job positions from pilot to air traffic control. He now resides in Iowa with his wife, Sheila, and dog, Tater.

He loves the outdoors and spends many hours on the rivers which run through Iowa.

He loves cooking and trying out new recipes, tweaking them to his taste with varying ingredients.

A music lover, he has played guitar since his teen years and continues his musical interest today with other instruments such as piano, hammered and mountain dulcimers.

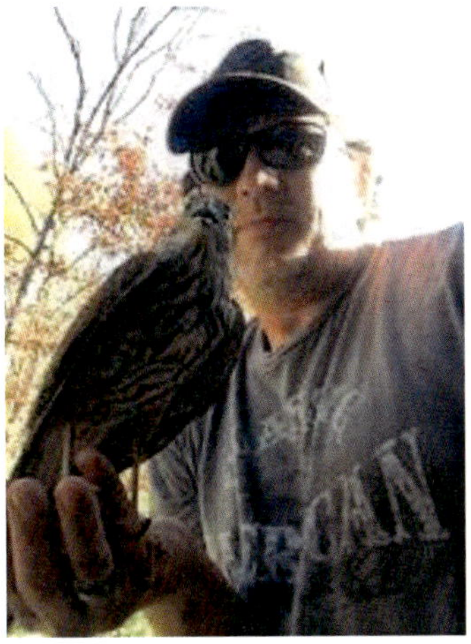

An avid animal lover, he is best known as the bird whisperer.

Joe loves hearing from his readers and would like to hear from you.

Have a recipe you want him to try? Send it to the address below. If it's selected for inclusion in his next recipe book entitled "The Best Recipes From Around the World," your name will appear as contributor for that recipe.

He can be reached at:

P.O. Box 4601
Des Moines, IA 50305